Radical Health

Radical Health

UNWELLNESS, CARE, AND LATINX EXPRESSIVE CULTURE

Julie Avril Minich

DUKE UNIVERSITY PRESS
Durham and London
2023

© 2023 DUKE UNIVERSITY PRESS
All rights reserved
Printed in the United States of America on acid-free paper ∞
Project Editor: Bird Williams
Designed by A. Mattson Gallagher
Typeset in Minion Pro by Westchester Publishing Services

Library of Congress Cataloging-in-Publication Data
Names: Minich, Julie Avril, [date] author.
Title: Radical health : unwellness, care, and Latinx expressive culture / Julie Avril Minich.
Description: Durham : Duke University Press, 2023. | Includes bibliographical references and index.
Identifiers: LCCN 2023001590 (print)
LCCN 2023001591 (ebook)
ISBN 9781478025252 (paperback)
ISBN 9781478020479 (hardcover)
ISBN 9781478027393 (ebook)
Subjects: LCSH: Hispanic Americans—Health and hygiene. | Hispanic Americans with disabilities. | Discrimination against people with disabilities—United States. | Health—Social aspects—United States. | Health services accessibility—United States. | Discrimination in medical care—United States. | Hispanic American arts—Social aspects. | Hispanic American arts—Political aspects. | BISAC: SOCIAL SCIENCE / People with Disabilities | HEALTH & FITNESS / Health Care Issues
Classification: LCC RA778.4.H57 M56 2023 (print) | LCC RA778.4.H57 (ebook) | DDC362.1089/68073—dc23/eng/20230527
LC record available at https://lccn.loc.gov/2023001590
LC ebook record available at https://lccn.loc.gov/2023001591

Cover art: Jaime Cortez, *Matriot* (2012). Charcoal on paper, 22 × 30 inches. Courtesy of the artist.

For Ignacio & Simón,
with love to Dominic

TABLE OF CONTENTS

ACKNOWLEDGMENTS

Radical Health was written on occupied land. I acknowledge in particular the Alabama-Coushatta, Caddo, Carrizo/Comecrudo, Coahuiltecan,
Comanche, Kickapoo, Lipan Apache, Tonkawa and Ysleta Del Sur Pueblo,
and all the American Indian and Indigenous Peoples and communities
who have been or have become a part of the lands and territories in central
Texas where I conducted most of the work for this book.

Over the many years it took me to write this book, the following enti-
ties provided financial support for my research and writing: the American
Council of Learned Societies Fellowship Program, the College of Liberal
Arts at the University of Texas at Austin (which provided both a College
Research Fellowship and a Humanities Research Award), and the Depart-
ments of English and Mexican American & Latina/o Studies at the University of Texas at Austin. The Department of Mexican American & Latina/o
Studies funded a manuscript workshop at a crucial stage in the writing of
this book; the critical and generous engagement I received at that workshop was absolutely invaluable. I am also grateful to my colleagues in the

Department of English, which hosted discussions of the first two chapters as work-in-progress talks, for their rigorous engagement with my work.

The following people have read extensive portions of the manuscript (in some cases, heroically, the entire thing) and offered inestimable insights: Karma R. Chávez, Ann Cvetkovich, Dominic Gonzales, Jennifer Harford Vargas, Rebeca L. Hey-Colón, Alison Kafer, Theresa A. Kulbaga, Jaimie Leanne Minich, Jasbir K. Puar, Ralph E. Rodríguez, Hershini Bhana Young, and three anonymous readers for Duke University Press. My editor at Duke University Press, Elizabeth Ault, was everything: patient when I needed it but also mindful of timing (and the paper shortages of the pandemic supply chain!); I'm especially grateful for her instinct for knowing exactly which readers the project needed. While the errors and inadequacies that remain are entirely mine, all of these sharp and generous individuals made this a much better book.

Audiences at talks I've given at the following institutions have also offered valuable engagement with the ideas in this book: Georgetown University; Michigan State University; Southwestern University; the University at Buffalo, State University of New York; the University of Houston; the University of Iowa; the University of Michigan–Ann Arbor; and the University of Wisconsin–Madison. I am grateful to Jennifer Natalya Fink, Alison Kafer, Karen Moroski-Rigney, Michael Rembis, Rene Rocha, Ariana Ruíz, Ellen Samuels, Sami Schalk, Alexandra Minna Stern, Jess Waggoner, Darrel Wanzer-Serrano, and Cynthia Wu for their labor in organizing these talks and accompanying events.

I am deeply grateful to my colleagues in the Department of English, the Department of Mexican American & Latina/o Studies, the Center for Mexican American Studies, and the Center for Women's and Gender Studies at the University of Texas at Austin for providing such an intellectually enriching place to work. Special thanks are due to the following UT colleagues: Frederick Luis Aldama, C. J. Álvarez, Minou Arjomand, Sam Baker, J. K. Barret, Phillip J. Barrish, Chad Bennett, Katy M. Buchanan, Luis Cárcamo-Huechante, Karma R. Chávez, Danielle Pilar Clealand, Cary Cordova, María Cotera, James H. Cox, T. Jackie Cuevas, Elizabeth Cullingford, Ann Cvetkovich (yes, Ann, I still consider you a UT colleague since your impact on this institution has made it the kind of place where I could thrive), Andrew Dell'Antonio, Liz Elsen, Caroline Faria, Richard R. Flores, Patricia M. García, John Morán González, Rachel V. González-Martin, Michael R. Hames-García, Luis Guevara, Jené Gutiérrez, Laura G. Gutiérrez, Susan S.

Heinzelman, Neville Hoad, Heather Houser, Grayson Hunt, Alison Kafer, Martin Kevorkian, Donna Kornhaber, Jeehyun Lim, Kelly McDonough, Lisa Lynn Moore, Gretchen Murphy, Lisa Olstein, Deborah Parra-Medina, Domino Renee Perez, Samantha Pinto, Elizabeth Richmond-Garza, Lilia Raquel Rosas, Jackie Salcedo, Patricia Schaub, Cathy J. Schlund-Vials, Ana Schwartz, Bassam Sidiki, Christen Smith, Cecilia Smith-Morris, Pauline T. Strong, Antonio Vásquez, Jennifer Wilks, and Hershini Bhana Young.

I am so lucky to have so many colleagues and friends beyond my institution. Too many people to possibly name here have supported me, so this is a partial list (which I attempted to alphabetize but may have erred): Ulka Anjaria, José Amador, Susan Antebi, Sony Coráñez Bolton, Deva Devika Bronson, Amy Sara Carroll, María Elena Cepeda, Mary Jean Corbett, Mayra Cortez-Cotto, Angie Cruz, Michael Cucher, John Alba Cutler, Micaela Díaz-Sánchez, Amanda Ellis, Julie Passanante Elman, Alex Espinoza, Elizabeth Freeman, Barbara Goodman, Richard Grijalva, Joshua Javier Guzmán, Monica Hanna, Emily Holmes, Jennifer James, Ronak K. Kapadia, Mimi Khúc, Jina B. Kim, Lawrence LaFountain, Travis Chi Wing Lau, Marisol Lebrón, Karlie Lemos, Brooke Lerner, Manuel López, Marissa López, Carmen Lugo-Lugo, Doris M. Madrigal, Ernesto Javier Martínez, Jorge Matos Valldejuli, Liza Mattison, John McKiernan-González, Marci McMahon, Robert McRuer, David Mitchell, Marisel Moreno, Paula M. L. Moya, Tamiko Nimura, Randy Ontiveros, Mariana Ortega, J Palmeri, Susan Pelle, Nina Perales, Gretchen Phillips, Therí Alyce Pickens, Andrea Pitts, Margaret Price, Jasbir K. Puar, Iván Ramos, John D. "Rio" Riofrio, Eliza Rodriguez, Ralph Rodriguez, Richard T. Rodríguez, Elda María Román, María Josefina Saldaña-Portillo, José David Saldívar, Ramón Saldívar, Ellen Samuels, Carmen Sanjuán-Pastor, Sami Schalk, Susan Schweik, Damon Scott, Tobin Siebers, Brittain Skinner, Melissa Spencer, Vanessa Torres, Margarita Urueña, David Vázquez, Dillon Vrana, Jess Waggoner, Sarah D. Wald, Priscilla Solis Ybarra, and Karla Zepeda. I'm lucky to have been friends with Amanda Lucas and Lydia Ruth Tietjen for three decades. Exchanges and collaborations with my *Crip Genealogies* coeditors (Mel Y. Chen, Alison Kafer, and Eunjung Kim) and with my Dis/color coeditors (Cynthia Wu and Nirmala Erevelles) also informed this project in crucial ways.

I could not do any of my work without artists. I'm so grateful to live in a world that still has art, and I wish to live in a world that supports artists better. The following artists, whether they are featured in this book or not, visited my classes and enriched my thinking while I was writing this book:

Virginia Grise, Caleb Luna, Jasminne Méndez, and ire'ne lara silva. Alynda Mariposa Segarra twice replied to my comments on Instagram, and I saw them perform live on four different occasions while writing this book.

Because of my amazing students, I've never believed that teaching takes time from research. In particular, the following students enriched my intellectual life while I was working on this book: Annie Bares, Pau Benavides, Audrey Berkemeier, Kim Canuette Grimaldi, John Carranza, Debbie Cifuentes Ramírez, José de la Garza-Valenzuela, Esther Díaz-Martin, Linda Eguiluz, Colleen Gleeson Eils, Sarai Flores, Stefanía García, Amanda Gray-Rendón, Alhelí Harvey, Roxana Loza, Caleb Luna, Brenda Martínez, Elizabeth (Libby) Martínez, Sneha Mehta, Regina Mills, Angie Núñez Rodríguez, Annyston Pennington, Lexi Pérez-Allison, Elena Pérez-Zetune, Lizzie Picherit, Rae Piwarski, Anahí Ponce, Michelle Rabe, Evan Rathjen, Weston Richey, Alexis Riley, Adena Rivera-Dundas, Mariana Rivera, Sarah Ropp, Ruth Rubio, Ipek Sahinler, Alexandra Salazar, Miriam Santana, Silvana Scott, Amanda Tovar, Daniel Vázquez Sanabria, Melissa Vera, and Brie Winnega.

While writing this book, I had many occasions to rage against my health insurance provider and the medical-industrial complex, but I remain deeply grateful to the health care workers who have made my own experience of health care less violent and more compassionate than it is for many. On confirming that I was unexpectedly pregnant, Sharon Liu matter-of-factly and nonjudgmentally gave me referrals to both an abortion provider and an ob-gyn; this is the kind of feminist health care everyone needs and deserves, and that is no longer available as of this writing to pregnant people who live in Texas. Crystal Berry-Roberts made me feel seen, heard, respected, and confident throughout a high-risk twin pregnancy and birth experience. My children's team of routine and specialized care providers, starting with Shai and Melissa in the NICU, whose full names I was too exhausted and terrified to learn but whose calming presence eased my stress tremendously, has been amazing. Special shout-outs go to pediatrician Katie Sanford and pediatric pulmonologist Ferdinand Coste.

This book would not have been written without the tireless and vastly undercompensated labor of childcare workers. I am especially grateful to Sara Brown, Lídice García, Roxana Jeréz, Izmirzi Medina, and Yolanda Tovar. Armandina Flores deserves special recognition for her tireless efforts to create a truly special place where my children and many others are loved and nurtured during uncertain times; while I was writing this book, she led the staff and families of our little school through a pandemic, a traumatic series of mass shootings, and a weather disaster that literally froze the entire state of Texas. I don't know how Ms. Dina and her team (including Ms. Alma and Mr. Jaime) do it all, but they are truly amazing!

Family makes us who we are, and I would not have written the book I did if I had a different family. I acknowledge my family in/around Georgia (Donna, David, Jaimie, Jonathan, Michelle, Joshua, Katie, Justin, Jonah, Conrad, Alice) and my family in Texas (Dominic, Louis, Oralia, Jeremy, Lilly, Ignacio, Simón). I love you all so much.

I am not adequate to the task of finding words that will convey how much the following people have enriched my life: my Best Feminists Forever (Kaidra L. Mitchell and Theresa A. Kulbaga), Alison Kafer, Jennifer Harford Vargas, Rebeca L. Hey-Colón, Jaimie Leanne Minich (the best sister in the universe), and Cynthia Wu.

Progress on this book would have proceeded much more expeditiously had it not been for the birth of my amazing children, Ignacio and Simón, but my life would have much less joy without them. I am so grateful to my children and to Dominic, my partner in life and in parenting, for all of the moments I spent with them that would otherwise have been spent on academic labor. My loves, this book is for you.

BOOK COVER DESCRIPTION: The image on the cover is a charcoal drawing by Jaime Cortez entitled *Matriot* (2012). The drawing is a black-and-white ambiguous image in which a dark silhouette forms a black shape with gray blood cells floating within it. This dark shape suggests the face in profile of a human skeleton, while the image formed by the white negative space appears as a standing feminine figure holding the hand of a child. The book title and name of the author are written in red over this negative white space. The book title–*Radical Health*–appears just beneath and to the right of the feminine figure, with a larger font than the rest of the text. The subtitle–*Unwellness, Care, and Latinx Expressive Culture*–is written into the body of the feminine figure. The author's name–Julie Avril Minich–appears at the bottom left, just beneath the body of a child.

Introduction

Radical Health/Radical Unwellness

On September 9, 2009, President Barack Obama addressed a joint session of Congress to introduce what would become his signature legislative achievement: the Patient Protection and Affordable Care Act (ACA). Knowing that he faced stiff opposition, Obama was careful to preempt his critics, declaring: "There are also those who claim that our reform effort will insure illegal immigrants. This, too, is false. The reforms—the reforms I'm proposing would not apply to those who are here illegally" (White House 2009). Representative Joe Wilson (R-SC), a critic of Obama's proposal, could not contain himself. "You lie!" he shouted in an extraordinary breach of congressional etiquette that drew national attention. Wilson was censured by the House of Representatives and forced to apologize (Hooper 2009), and his outburst has been remembered as both an effort to sow disinformation and an expression of white resentment toward the first Black president of the United States. However, these characterizations—accurate as they are—miss another important truth: Wilson and Obama *agreed* on the exclusion of undocumented immigrants from a national health care plan (and coincided in their use of the pejorative descriptor *illegal*). Both Obama's speech and Wilson's response thus demonstrate how anxieties about race and citizenship saturate national conversations about health care.

Five years after the ACA's passage, the arrest of Blanca Borrego demonstrates the cost of Obama's acquiescence to anti-immigrant sentiment. On September 3, 2015, Borrego went to an appointment at the new office of her longtime gynecologist and presented proof of insurance through her spouse's employer. Asked for identification, Borrego (who was undocumented) offered a fake driver's license. She was then taken to an exam room where she was arrested by a sheriff's deputy who escorted her out of the facility (Schiller 2015). The fact that a health care worker felt compelled to call law enforcement on a woman seeking medical treatment using private insurance reveals the stakes of debates over who should—and should not—access care.

Borrego's entire family felt the impact of her arrest: her spouse quit his job in fear of deportation, while her teenage son (who had a work permit through the Deferred Action for Childhood Arrivals, or DACA, program) became the family's sole wage earner. Likewise, measures to terrorize undocumented immigrants reverberate throughout Latinx communities. In part this is because many Latinx people, like Borrego, belong to mixed-status families, but it is also (and more importantly) because the figure of the undocumented immigrant is a crucial rhetorical device in the racialization of Latinx people. Historians have demonstrated that immigration restrictions and border enforcement are not simply the result of racist biases but are mutually constituted with them (Hernandez 2010; Lew-Williams 2018; Martinez 2018; Molina 2014; Ngai 2004).[1] To understand the racialization of Latinx communities as intertwined with anti-immigrant sentiment, then, is not to conflate the categories of "Latinx" and "immigrant"—or even to suggest that all Latinx people identify with or as immigrants—but rather to note the critical function of anti-immigrant discourse in the social construction of Latinidad more broadly.

Yet even as Borrego's family and community felt the effects of her arrest, they also mobilized in response. As her son supported the family on a waiter's pay, Borrego's daughter took to the media in protest: "My mom is a good person. . . . She doesn't deserve what's going on" (Garcia-Ditta 2015). Like Borrego's daughter, Latinx cultural workers—writers, filmmakers, musicians, performers, visual artists—create narratives that counter the messages of a xenophobic and white supremacist national culture. This book focuses on one subset of this cultural production: art (especially literature) addressing the relationship between Latinx communities and the health care system, advancing an ethic of radical health that embraces racialized, disabled, and otherwise devalued bodyminds.[2]

Why Health?

Radical Health: Unwellness, Care, and Latinx Expressive Culture argues that Latinx expressive culture can offer a powerful intervention in contemporary US health politics. First, it elaborates how certain Latinx artists expose ideologies of health as an engine of racism, following geographer Ruth Wilson Gilmore's famous definition of racism as "the state-sanctioned or extralegal production and exploitation of group-differentiated vulnerability to premature death" (2007, 28). In particular, I trace how these cultural workers critique notions of health as the result of personal behavior that render Latinx communities *radically unwell* by eliding structural determinants of health. Second, and more importantly, I explore the politics of *radical health* emerging from cultural artifacts that present health not as individual duty but as communal responsibility. This latter thread of my argument, which constitutes the bulk of my analysis, examines texts by Latinx artists who seek to elucidate the collective and societal aspects of wellbeing, presenting health as a political concern rather than a purely individual, medical one. Here I claim a role for artistic work and cultural studies scholarship in the effort to combat both health stigma and racial health disparities.

I use the word *radical* throughout this study to emphasize that my focus is not on *reforming* health care but rather on fundamentally *reimagining* what health means and how health resources are distributed. I use the word *health* to signal my commitment to the field of disability studies as well as to clarify my position within it. Disability studies, as Jina B. Kim has observed, partially owes its urgency to the fact that, in the contemporary United States, "disability, debility, and illness have emerged as primary arenas for racialized punishment" (2020, 266). At the same time, a tendency among scholars in the field to reject (rather than critically engage with) discourses of health, cure, and medicalization can leave it poorly equipped to address this concern.[3] In fact, Black feminists Moya Bailey and Izetta Autumn Mobley highlight the long-standing critique by disability scholars of medical models of disability as one of the field's major barriers to advancing racial justice: "While certainly the medical model is a problematic trope, it may signal differently to communities that have tried for many decades to receive the most elementary care only to be refused. As uncomfortable as it may make those of us engaged in the Disability Studies field, some communities are actually yearning for not only care but treatment and cure" (2019, 28). In titling this book *Radical Health,* I posit that a reassessment of health can contribute to what Kim (2017, 2021) calls a crip-of-color critique and what Sami Schalk and Kim (2020) call a feminist-of-color disability studies, terms that signal the need for scholarship that is both anti-ableist and anti-racist.

Crip-of-color critique is not merely a subset of disability studies that combines perspectives from ethnic studies with the insights of disability theory; it is a substantially new body of knowledge that reexamines what disability is, what disability studies does, and who disability theory is for. In other words, rather than merely diversifying the field or unsettling its long-acknowledged whiteness, crip-of-color critique remakes disability studies. The intellectual precursors to crip-of-color critique emerge not solely from disability studies but also from critical race studies, and most importantly from Black studies. For instance, the term *crip-of-color critique* is not simply a clever restatement of Roderick A. Ferguson's now-famous phrase *queer-of-color critique,* but rather an extension of Ferguson's effort to debunk "the idea that race, class, gender, and sexuality are discrete formations, apparently insulated from one another" (2004, 4), and to identify processes of racialization within cultural formations that present themselves as unrelated to race. Schalk and Kim insist that critical race theories must "inform work in disability studies as a whole even when people of color are absent as sites of analysis" (2020, 33). Similarly, Sony Coráñez Bolton (2023) has made the provocative move of claiming that the focus on colonized embodiment within Filipinx studies constitutes it as a mode of crip theorizing. Although the term *crip-of-color critique* is relatively new in the disability studies lexicon, the insistence that a focus on race and racialization fundamentally changes the field is not. In a foundational special issue of *MELUS* on race and disability, Jennifer C. James and Cynthia Wu urge disability scholars to consider "how disability has always been racialized, gendered, and classed and how racial, gender, and class difference have been conceived of as 'disability'" (2006, 8). At the same time, and more pointedly, Chris Bell suggests that a disability studies intent on equating "visibility with inclusivity" (2006, 279)—that is, citing examples of disabled activists and scholars of color without committing to the intersectional analysis they demand—might more accurately be named white disability studies.

While disability studies scholars often locate the origins of the field in disability rights activism, scholars who align their work with crip-of-color critique often look as well to activist work in which disability does not always present as the primary concern. In describing the activism that informs her theory of Black disability politics, for instance, Schalk notes that "the articulation and enactment of Black disability politics do not necessarily center traditional disability rights language and approaches, such as disability pride or civil rights inclusion, instead prioritizing an understanding of disability within the context of white supremacy" (2022, 5). Rather than disability *rights*, crip-of-color critique often emphasizes disability *justice*. As Mia Mingus (2011) defines it, disability justice means "moving away from an equality-based model of sameness and 'we are just like you' to a model of disability that embraces difference, confronts privilege and challenges what is considered 'normal' on every front." For Patty Berne (2015), a "Disability Justice framework understands that all bodies are . . . caught in these bindings of ability, race, gender, sexuality, class, nation state and imperialism, and that we cannot separate them." The activism that forms the theoretical base of crip-of-color critique, then, centers not just disability but multiple and mutually reinforcing systems of oppression; the embrace of interdependence over independence; and the desire for revolution over reform.

A survey of twentieth-century Latinx history demonstrates how ideologies of health and ability have shaped the social and political construction of Latinx identities and the racialization of Latinx people. For instance, 1904's *Gonzales v. Williams*, the US Supreme Court case that established Puerto Ricans as "noncitizen nationals" and set the legal precedent for the second-class citizenship that Puerto Ricans still experience, was set in motion when immigration inspectors at Ellis Island noticed the visible pregnancy of Isabel González, deemed her "likely to become a public charge," and placed her in detention (Erman 2019). Latinx history offers a record of how disability and health affect the US immigration system as well as how that system affects the bodies of migrants: Alexandra Minna Stern (1999), Natalia Molina (2006), and John McKiernan-González (2012) detail how Latinx migrants have been treated as vectors of disease, while Mary E. Mendoza (2017) and Seth Holmes (2013) demonstrate the debilitating living and working conditions that Latinx agricultural workers experience. Eugenic ideologies of health, meanwhile, subject Latinx people regardless of citizenship status to coercive sterilizations and reproductive abuse, as Laura Briggs (2003), Elena R. Gutiérrez (2008), and Natalie Lira (2021) show.

Responding to these histories, Latinx struggles for racial justice have often been organized around concerns of health and wellbeing. The activism of César Chávez for the health and wellbeing of agricultural workers is memorialized in a national monument, a major motion picture, and the street names of several major US cities, but the health advocacy of the New York Young Lords, which organized hospital takeovers, offered testing for tuberculosis and lead exposure, and staged a Garbage Offensive to protest discriminatory city sanitation services, also merits close attention (Fernández 2020; Morales 2016; Wanzer-Serrano 2015). Schalk and Kim argue that such activist work should not be seen merely as an underrepresented object of analysis in disability studies but should be treated as an unacknowledged contribution to disability theory because it produces new knowledge about the intersection of race, gender, and ability.[4]

This study begins with texts published in the mid-1990s and extends to the contemporary period. In the United States, this period saw expanded opportunities for people with disabilities to participate in public life, a significant retraction of the social safety net, and vociferous debates over immigration policy—all of which come to bear on current public discourse related to the US health care system. The writers and artists whose work I examine reflect these social conditions in their work through their inclusive representations of diverse bodyminds, their concern for how ideologies of individual self-reliance prevent vulnerable people from accessing care and support, and their direct engagement with the consequences of border enforcement. The texts I analyze in this book thus capture and respond to these national conversations, offering not policy analysis but aesthetic renderings of the relationship between personal wellbeing and social climate. In particular, three laws from the 1980s and 1990s shape the political environment from which these texts emerge: the 1986 Immigration Reform and Control Act (IRCA), which formalized the status of approximately three million undocumented residents of the United States and created new immigration control infrastructure; the 1990 Americans with Disabilities Act (ADA), which prohibited disability discrimination and guaranteed employment and educational opportunities for people with disabilities; and the 1996 Personal Responsibility and Work Opportunity Reconciliation Act (PRWORA), which (as President Bill Clinton proudly proclaimed) "ended welfare as we knew it." None of the texts I examine in this book directly mentions these laws by name, but they all respond to (and in some instances capitulate to) a social climate marked by scrutiny and resentment directed toward people who access increasingly scarce public resources and by the sense that people's wellbeing is a matter of personal (rather than public or collective) responsibility.

The first two laws, signed by Republican presidents, seem to enact policies to the left of the current political center in the United States; the latter, signed by a Democrat, constitutes the kind of decimation of safety nets typically attributed to politicians on the right. (Together, these laws demonstrate how far to the right both US political parties have moved in the past half-century.) The IRCA, for instance, has been retrospectively characterized as an "amnesty program" but also spurred anti-immigrant backlash (Abrajano and Hajnal 2015). Meanwhile, the ADA secured the right to work for disabled people but not the right *not* to work; as Sunny Taylor (2004) reminds us, it reinforced the idea that people with disabilities should seek employment rather than relying on public benefits.[5] Finally, PRWORA both institutionalized the notion of "personal responsibility" that has figured so prominently in debates over the ACA and exacerbated the need for health care reform by severely limiting Medicaid eligibility.[6] Public debates about these laws echo in those surrounding the ACA, which in addition to presenting the undocumented as unworthy of health care also reinforce the idea that people forced to rely on the state for life-sustaining resources are irresponsible and undeserving. For instance, during a 2017 push to repeal the ACA, Representative Jason Chaffetz (R-UT) suggested that the reason many people could not afford health care was their smartphone purchases: "Americans have choices," he told CNN. "And they've got to make a choice. And so, maybe rather than getting that new iPhone that they just love and they want to go spend hundreds of dollars on that, maybe they should invest it in their own health care."[7]

I rehearse this history because, as I finish writing this book in the immediate aftermath of Donald Trump's White House occupancy and the ongoing devastation of the COVID-19 pandemic, it feels urgent to remember that this moment, while dire, is not exceptional. I began this book in 2014, the year most provisions of the ACA came into effect. At that time, I held an unequivocally critical stance toward the law: I considered its exclusion of undocumented immigrants both morally reprehensible and bad public health practice, and I opposed as well its promotion of an individualist approach to health.[8] By the time I finished my first draft of this manuscript, things had changed dramatically. It was 2020, more than three years into Trump's time in the White House; the future of the ACA was (and is) uncertain; increasingly draconian policies were being enacted against immigrants; and debates about public health measures to curb the spread of COVID-19 were fiercely underway. Indeed, in the context of the COVID-19 pandemic, the idea of health as an individual responsibility has turned deadly, with a prominent and vocal minority of the US population loudly and violently asserting its right to refuse public health precautions and endanger the lives of others. This book, then, which began as a polemic against the ACA, became an effort to expose and dismantle the racial animus that undergirds national conversations about public health and to illuminate how Latinx cultural workers have reimagined health and wellbeing.

Radical Health thus treats the work of contemporary Latinx cultural workers as a source of theoretical insight about disability, health, and wellbeing. It tells the stories not of the twentieth-century social actors, like Isabel González or the Young Lords, who contested racializing discourses of health and racial health disparities, but of contemporary Latinx cultural workers who have demanded access to health resources even as they have also sought to redefine health itself. My use of the phrase *radical health* captures how these cultural workers advance a critique of health (as a punitive ideology used to devalue and disparage people whose bodily practices do not conform to social norms) even as they seek to claim it.

Health as Racializing Ideology

To illuminate how the texts I study reimagine health, I first address the ideological function of health as an instrument of racialization. The aforementioned debates about the passage and implementation of the ACA are a useful starting point both because of the ACA's exclusion of undocumented immigrants and because of what these debates reveal about who is understood to deserve health and who is not. I am not, of course, the first to criticize the ACA, a law that historian Colin Gordon (2018) calls a "spectacularly imperfect solution to our healthcare crisis." There are many good critiques of the ACA; mine focuses on the law's designation of particular people as ineligible.[9] The narrative that some people simply *had* to be excluded for the ACA to pass reifies the idea that the health of the nation depends on withholding health from certain populations.[10] Of course, this idea is patently false. Health is not a finite resource that grows scarcer as it is made more widely available. If the COVID-19 crisis has taught us anything, it is that the *more* people within a community have access to health resources—including not just doctors and medicines but also paid sick leave, safe childcare, food security, and safe housing—the healthier everyone in that community can be. In an earlier assessment of the repeated failures to create a national health care plan in the twentieth-century United States,

Gordon (2003) faults not the overreach of activists who attempted to cover too many people (as common explanations have it) but reformers' willingness to compromise and leave people out. By accepting certain exclusions as necessary, advocates of "universal" health care affirmed "distinctions between deserving and undeserving citizens" (9), undermining not only their cause but public health itself. By declaring from the outset that undocumented people would be ineligible for benefits, advocates of the ACA effectively opened the door to further discussion of whether certain categories of people deserve health care at all—a conversation that has left the law itself precarious.

The flaws of a health care system that denies care to entire populations came dramatically to light in 2020 with the spread of COVID-19, even as the pandemic also laid bare the impulse to blame under-resourced populations for their poor health outcomes. In the United States, for instance, death rates in Black and Latinx communities have been blamed on comorbidities resulting from "unhealthy" lifestyles (like fatness and diabetes), rather than on unequal health care access, on the overrepresentation of Black and Latinx people among the essential workers most exposed to the coronavirus that causes COVID-19, or on patterns of residential discrimination that concentrate Black and Latinx people into high-density dwellings where social distancing is difficult. Meanwhile, once a COVID-19 vaccine became available, the (initially) lower vaccination rates in Black and Latinx communities were immediately attributed to vaccine hesitancy rather than to lack of access. When vaccines in the United States were in short supply, debates raged about whether certain categories of people (including fat people, smokers, and undocumented immigrants) should receive them, suggesting a widespread belief that certain people deserved to die of a preventable illness. Once the vaccines became widely available, vaccine mandates were framed as an imposition on healthy people, whose personal freedom to refuse vaccination was valorized above the lives of the vulnerable people that universal vaccination would protect. The toll of the COVID-19 pandemic—and the ways in which racialized death was normalized and rationalized—reinforces a pointed critique of the US health care system by the disability scholar Nirmala Erevelles: "Why do some bodies matter more than others?" (2011, 6).

The idea that personal behaviors or beliefs are the primary cause of health disparities is linked to what the sociologist Robert Crawford calls *healthism*: "the ideology of individual responsibility for health" (1980, 367).[11] To be perceived as deserving health in a society that embraces healthism, one must care for one's body according to very precise social norms: avoiding tobacco and other controlled substances, eating a diet deemed nutritious, wearing sunscreen, refusing to engage in risky sex practices, and exercising often. Meanwhile, those seen as undeserving often experience bodily conditions, erroneously believed to result solely from irresponsible personal choices, that have a disproportionately adverse effect in communities of color and among people of lower socioeconomic status: fatness, asthma, diabetes, sexually transmitted infections, addiction, high-risk or stigmatized pregnancies, mental illness, and some cancers and neurological differences.[12] Healthism pervades the political rhetoric of liberals and conservatives alike; it surfaces in Republican efforts to dismantle the ACA as well as in local ordinances (many sponsored by Democrats) banning the construction of new fast-food restaurants or dollar stores, out of the belief that such establishments promote "bad" food choices among the poor (Capelouto 2019; Chandler 2015; Ward 2013). It is not, I believe, coincidental that Obama, the president who finally did expand health care access, was tall, normatively attractive, and personally invested in performing health (he took pains to conceal his cigarette addiction and highlight his time on the basketball court when he moved into the White House)—nor do I think it coincidental that the signature charitable cause of his spouse, Michelle Obama, was an effort called *Let's Move!* focused on individual health behaviors like exercise and the consumption of fresh, unprocessed foods.[13]

The notion that people are personally responsible for their own health also aligns with an idea long critiqued by disability scholars: what Robert McRuer (2006) calls *compulsory able-bodiedness*. McRuer defines compulsory able-bodiedness as the commonsense agreement that "able-bodied identities, able-bodied perspectives are preferable and what we all, collectively, are aiming for" (9). Compulsory able-bodiedness is often understood to describe the demand that people perform to their maximum ability at all times (taking the stairs instead of the elevator, even if it means exhaustion later; refusing necessary accommodations at work or at school to avoid the appearance of "preferential treatment," etc.) and the emphasis of charities promoting the "search for a cure" rather than improvements to the quality of life for people with disabilities. But compulsory able-bodiedness is also at work in the mandate to protect one's health at all times and at all costs. Under a system of compulsory able-bodiedness, behaviors that might foster a sense of wellbeing but are not considered "healthy" (like eating a piece of cake, smoking a joint, or having anonymous sex) are subject to shaming and punishment. Those unable or unwilling to consistently perform normative health behaviors are seen not merely as responsible for their own ill health but as a burden on society, a drain on valuable resources, unworthy of care or protection, and ultimately disposable.

Radical Health interrogates how healthism and compulsory able-bodiedness justify the health disparities that affect Latinx communities. While the case of Blanca Borrego, criminalized for seeking medical care, represents the overt denial of care to Latinx people, healthism and compulsory able-bodiedness are more insidious: they present health concerns affecting Latinx communities, from HIV/AIDS to diabetes, as the result of pathologized personal behaviors or cultural attributes rather than structural inequities. There are echoes here of what the historian Alan M. Kraut calls "medicalized nativism" (1994, 3). Medicalized nativism, as Priscilla Wald observes, "involves more than superimposing a disease threat on an unfortunate group" (2008, 8); it also links disease to "dangerous practices and behaviors that allegedly mark intrinsic cultural difference" and that express "the destructive transformative power of the group" (8). *Radical Health* begins at the intersection of medicalized nativism with neoliberal notions of individual responsibility, where the "dangerous practices and behaviors" attributed to Latinx people are used to explain the health concerns affecting their communities and where racialized health disparities become an argument against (rather than for) universal health care.

Dominant ideas about health are not merely the result of racial bias; they can foment white supremacy. Sociologist Eduardo Bonilla-Silva identifies "the curious enigma of 'racism without racists'" (2014, 4), a phenomenon in which purportedly race-neutral policies and ideologies produce racially unequal outcomes.[14] Health, I argue, is one apparently race-neutral ideology that perpetuates racial inequality. When poor health is understood as the result of bad personal choices and not the systemic denial of access to health-sustaining resources, then entire communities are blamed for their illnesses, impairments, and deaths. Furthermore, when health is construed as the result of good personal choices (motivation, restraint, discipline), those experiencing illness are constructed as indolent, gluttonous, and negligent—adjectives with a long history in racializing discourse. In this way, health can function as both an outcome and a source of racial injustice. Therefore, while the phenomenon of "racism without racists" described by Bonilla-Silva operates across numerous sites, *health* is a particularly important one—and one that I believe has been underexamined as a key theme in Latinx aesthetic representations.

Radical Health

Against the racializing ideologies of health just described, this book examines the work of Latinx artists advancing a politics of radical health. I define *radical health* as a vision of health that simultaneously emphasizes its structural dimensions and refuses to treat it as a measure of human worth. Here I offer two distinct—even at times incongruous—lines of analysis. First, I address how Latinx expressive culture makes visible the context in which people make health decisions. In response to healthism, compulsory ablebodiedness, and the neoliberal policies they promote, the texts examined in the following chapters reveal factors beyond individual control—access to nutritious food, medical care and information, clean air and water, and cultural representations portraying one's life as valuable and worth living—that affect physical and mental wellbeing. Second, I emphasize how the texts I study present the value of Latinx lives independently of health status. These texts depict people who are HIV-positive, fat, diabetic, and otherwise labeled as unhealthy in ways that reject the stigma of unhealth. Latina fat activist Virgie Tovar (2015) exemplifies this latter strategy: "There are . . . those whose politics align largely with my own who are committed to pleading a case that my body is a failure that is 'not my fault.' . . . But I'm not interested in exonerating myself. And perhaps more importantly, there is nothing that needs exonerating." From this angle, one might note that this book could just as easily be titled *Radical Unwellness* (which was, in fact, one of my early working titles), since some of the texts I examine offer such sharp critiques of the conflation of a person's social value with their health status that they can be read as an embrace of unhealth. Ultimately, however, I chose to put the word *health* in my title not to reaffirm its value but to signal my commitment to interrogating it.

At first glance, the fact that so many of the artists I study simultaneously critique the structural factors that lead to racial health disparities *and* celebrate the bodies shaped by these disparities might seem contradictory or even incoherent (and, as my discussion of individual texts will show, contradictions and incoherencies do arise). These contradictions, however, illuminate a larger theoretical conundrum. As crip theorist Alison Kafer asks: "How can we attend to 'serious health problems' while also deconstructing the stigma attached to those problems or even historicizing the very construction of such conditions as problems?" (2013, 159). Kafer's question is motivated by an effort to find coalition between disability and environmental justice activists, but given the systemic denial of health care to poor people of color, it has much wider implications. Answering Kafer's question requires nuancing disability rights discourses that celebrate nonnormative bodies without critiquing the social conditions that produce them. Jasbir K. Puar, for instance, notes the limitations of disability scholarship and activism that is singularly focused on reclamation: "In a context whereby four-fifths of the world's people with disabilities are located in what was once hailed as the 'global south,' liberal interventions are invariably infused with certitude that disability should be reclaimed as a valuable difference—the difference of the Other—through rights, visibility, and empowerment discourses—rather than addressing how much debilitation is caused by global injustice and the war machines of colonialism, occupation, and U.S. imperialism" (2017, xvii). Erevelles pointedly asks: "How is disability celebrated if its very existence is inextricably linked to the violence of social/economic conditions of capitalism?" (2011, 17). And while the tension between disability pride and the effort to address health injustice may lack a definitive resolution, I believe it is urgent to work from that tension in a political moment when communities of color and the poor are uniquely vulnerable to disease and impairment even as such communities are collectively blamed and stigmatized for their ill health. This book therefore centers the work of artists who embrace debilitated bodies while critiquing systems of debilitation.

Although my methods are primarily those of the literary critic, I have found that attending to the vision of radical health offered by the texts discussed in this study requires citing scholars from outside literary studies as much as scholars from within it. Like literary critics Paula M. L. Moya and John Alba Cutler, I understand literary scholarship as fundamentally and necessarily in conversation with the work of other disciplines, particularly the social sciences, and I understand art of all kinds as an endeavor that is both aesthetic and ideological. In different contexts, Moya and Cutler have both demonstrated how the methods of literary criticism—including close reading, formal analysis, and theoretical engagement—serve as an intervention into pressing social concerns. Moya asserts that literary criticism has a necessarily sociopolitical dimension, as a "close reading of a work of literature can . . . serve as an excavation of, and a meditation on, the pervasive sociocultural ideas—such as race, ethnicity, gender, and sexuality—of the social worlds . . . within which both authors and readers live" (2016, 8–9). Cutler, meanwhile, argues that the work of social scientists is often more literary than acknowledged; within it, our social world "is never simply observed—it is produced and reproduced" (2015, 8).

In addition to drawing from literary studies, critical ethnic studies, and crip-of-color critique, I take inspiration from the rejection of respectability politics that characterizes queer-of-color critique. Respectability politics, as Juana María Rodríguez notes, allege "that in order to enter the fold of collectivity, be it familial or revolutionary, we must first be liberated of our sexual deviance and our politically incorrect desires" (2014, 11). Like Rodríguez, I am interested in bodyminds that "exceed the norms of proper corporeal containment" (2014, 2), but where Rodríguez focuses on the eruption of bodily excess in sexual practice, *Radical Health* examines it in medical scenarios, where the "politically incorrect desires" precluding entrance into the collectivity might include simple carbohydrates or sex without condoms (however vanilla that sex might otherwise be). As Lisa Marie Cacho observes: "Ascribing readily recognizable social value always requires the devaluation of an/other, and that other is almost always poor, racialized, criminalized, segregated, legally vulnerable, and unprotected" (2012, 17). To Cacho's list of devalued others I add the *radically unwell*: the diseased, the disabled, the unhealthy, and the debilitated.

One salient example of how the effort to claim the value of some can devalue others is visible in some public health scholarship emphasizing the Latinx Health Paradox. Also known as the Hispanic Health Paradox and the Healthy Latino Paradox, this concept describes a phenomenon observed by public health researchers that Latinx immigrant populations tend to have better health outcomes than their socioeconomic status would predict. As originally theorized by the sociologist Rubén G. Rumbaut, the Latinx Health Paradox seems at first glance to challenge the "ethnocentric assumptions" (1997, 490) that position immigrants from Latin America as a burden on the US health care system. Yet there are reasons to be cautious about characterizing Latinx communities as "a super-healthy population with differing health promotion and services needs" (Vega and Amaro 1994, 40). Medical anthropologist Seth Holmes (2013) notes the vast intra-ethnic diversity within the category "Latinx" and observes specifically that migrant and seasonal agricultural workers—a category in which immigrants from Mexico and Central America are overrepresented—experience much poorer health status than nearly all other workers. And, most relevant to my argument, many researchers have noted that the Latinx Health Paradox relies on essentializing notions of culture and ignores structural factors that influence health (Castañeda et al. 2015; Viruell-Fuentes, Miranda, and Abdulrahim 2012). Scholars who invoke the Latinx Health Paradox tend to speculate about behaviors linked to cultural belief systems that offer health benefits, but, as Edna A. Viruell-Fuentes argues, this approach "runs the risk of lending support to victim-blaming explanations for health outcomes" since the "idea of culture as a 'source of dysfunction' can easily flow from this line of thinking" (2007, 1525). The problems of leaning too heavily on discourses like the Latinx Health Paradox are also made visible in scholarship from adjacent fields, particularly Asian American studies scholarship examining the role of health in constructing a "model minority" identity (Lee 2021; Shah 2001).

Just as the focus on health distinguishes *Radical Health* from disability scholarship that takes a purely critical stance toward healing and cure, so too does my emphasis on crip-of-color critique differentiate this study from literary criticism rooted in a medical humanities approach known as narrative medicine. Developed by the physician-scholar Rita Charon, narrative medicine refers to "medicine practiced with these narrative skills of recognizing, absorbing, interpreting, and being moved by stories of illness" (2006, 3). While I share Charon's interest in the subjective experience of health and unwellness, and applaud her efforts to integrate narrative theory into medical education, I believe that cultural texts have more to offer than the fostering of individualized compassion, empathy, and care; in addition, they offer a means of imagining our social world otherwise and a proposal for structural change.[15]

The texts examined in this book engage with health on both individual and structural levels, making visible the larger context in which people make health decisions but also revealing people's individual (sometimes imperfect, always complicated) navigation of structural constraints. While the task of the social scientist is to note and describe this navigation, the task of the artist is to show us what it looks and feels like in practice, undertaken by people with messy desires, limitations, and flaws. Because the sustained analysis of cultural artifacts requires a simultaneous examination of both individual behaviors *and* larger systems, cultural criticism is an important resource for understanding health disparities. This is especially true because the individual threads of an argument in cultural studies scholarship don't always align perfectly: different artists approach social concerns differently, and even a singular artwork may be characterized by internal incongruities whose convolutions mirror those of the thorny social issues it navigates. Thus, having elaborated my argument, I now turn to a work of art that illuminates the tensions within it: the performance manifesto *Your Healing Is Killing Me* by Chicana playwright and performance artist Virginia Grise.

PAUSE: Virginia Grise, *Your Healing Is Killing Me*

Your Healing Is Killing Me (YHIKM) follows the journey of an artist with severe eczema to find relief from her symptoms. As a chronic condition of unknown cause, linked to genetics but triggered by environmental factors and stress, eczema prompts the speaker to meditate on both the injustices of a capitalist health care system and the intergenerational PTSD (caused by migration, war, and sexual violence) that affects her family. The text, in other words, substantiates a lament from disability justice activist Leah Lakshmi Piepzna-Samarasinha: "Everyone I know longs for healing. It's just hard to get. The good kind of healing: healing that is affordable, has child-care and no stairs, doesn't misgender us or disrespect our disabilities or sex work, believes us when we're hurt and listens when we say what we need, understands that we are the first and last authorities on our own bodies and minds" (2018, 97–98). YHIKM layers the speaker's current life as a working artist with memories of childhood trauma and experiences with healers from *curanderas* to acupuncturists to dermatologists, showing that finding the "good kind of healing" requires her to address not just one physical ailment but longer histories: neoliberal economic policies that curtail possibilities of social mobility, making survival as a working artist tenuous; the Vietnam War and its effect on her father's mental health; her mother's and sisters' migrations between Mexico and the United States; and her childhood experiences with sexual violence. The speaker tries numerous treatments, some of which help temporarily and many of which create new problems (like the steroid cream that induces dependency, rapid weight loss, and mood swings).

In addition to moving between personal and structural registers, YHIKM also engages the complexity of what Eunjung Kim (2017) calls "curative violence." The text contains a staunch critique of capitalist influences in the health care system, detailing the barriers to treatment faced by a working artist with no health insurance, but its emphasis on finding a cure for the speaker's eczema also places it in tension with what activist Eli Clare calls the "anti-cure politics" (2017, 60) of the mainstream disability movement. Another potential concern for some might be the treatment that the speaker ultimately finds for her eczema—bone soup, cooked weekly by her lover: "Bone soup builds immunity, helps with inflammation and digestion. Some say it even fights cancer. After all those visits to the nice lady doctor and the fancy dermatologist and the cynical acupuncturist, I found out that what I needed was right in my kitchen the whole time" (Grise 2017, 82). While the fact that the speaker finds a treatment option outside of a capitalist health industry drives home the critique of profit-driven health care, the experience of receiving invasive and patronizing health recommendations (often in the form of "holistic" medicines or dietary changes) from well-meaning strangers is a common and frustrating experience for many people with disabilities and chronic illnesses. In other words, despite its benefits to the speaker of this particular text, bone soup may be as ineffective and harmful for some chronically ill people as for-profit medicine.

Yet as the speaker of YHIKM delves into the possible causes of and treatments for her eczema, she ultimately arrives at an exhaustive list of things that are killing her (that is, not only worsening her eczema but shortening her life), a list that covers medicine, the health care system, food production and distribution systems, economic inequality, white supremacy, the lack of a viable political left in the United States, gender roles, and more. While the desire for relief that permeates YHIKM and the cure that results might sit uneasily with some disability scholars and activists, Grise's delicate negotiation of the need to balance critique of the health care system with investment in healing places her work firmly in conversation with scholars and activists like Eli Clare and Eunjung Kim, who seek to complicate how disability communities engage with cure.

It is important, then, to note that although the *plot* of YHIKM ends with a cure, the *text* does not. Here I refer back to my earlier point that while the plot of YHIKM follows the speaker's journey to find relief for eczema symptoms, the monologues that make up the manifesto tell a comprehensive story of the speaker's experiences with trauma, illness, and healing. After sharing her experience with relief from her symptoms via bone soup, the speaker offers a proclamation suggesting that even if *she* has found a solution that works for her, the structural problems that exacerbated her eczema remain intact:

> Capitalism is toxic. No amount of body butter or eczema creams will act as a salve for its toxicity. As a system it cannot be fixed. The only way to defend ourselves against it is to destroy it. The only way to destroy it is to create something better. In the process, we must be willing to assess, to prepare, to study, to fight, but we must also be willing to listen to ourselves and each other, to change, to transform, to care for ourselves and each other. . . .
>
> I am an artist. And as an artist, I believe that my greatest creative project is to imagine something, something better, where our dreams matter, where as a people we are free. (Grise 2017, 83)

This conclusion prompts spectators to understand health and wellbeing as concerns that demand political solutions even when individual symptoms are resolved. YHIKM further makes a claim for *art* as the medium through which people are able to imagine better ways of ensuring each other's wellbeing. While the writers and artists discussed throughout this book differ in their assessments of the health care system, the kinds of bodily conditions they address, and their strategies for combating the stigma of unwellness, their work is united by the effort to make an aesthetic, imaginative argument for a politics of radical health.

Latinx Expressive Culture (or "Latino Is Not a Politic")

My engagement with Grise in the previous section requires that I end this introduction with some final comments about why I have specifically located my exploration of radical health in a group of interpretive objects that I label as *Latinx expressive culture*—a category that, as much recent scholarship demonstrates, merits some pressure. In fact, in YHIKM, Grise's speaker pointedly rejects *Latinx* as a basis for collective action (and, implicitly, as a basis for collective aesthetics as well), asserting that "Pan-Latino(ism) is killing me, as Latino is not a politic nor an ideology and does nothing to prepare us to defend ourselves against what is actually killing us" (2017, 57). Indeed, although I argue that a conceptualization of radical health comes into focus from the collective analysis of a range of contemporary Latinx cultural artifacts, not only do I seek to avoid imposing ideological uniformity on the texts I examine, I want to be clear that I don't even love (or agree with) them all equally. As just one salient example of the dissonance that surfaces between the writers and artists I discuss, chapter 2 (on diabetic representation) juxtaposes a piece coauthored by Grise, a committed prison abolitionist, against an autobiography by Supreme Court Justice Sonia Sotomayor, who began her career as a prosecutor. Of course, Latinx studies as a field has always understood Latinidad as what the political theorist Cristina Beltrán calls "a site of permanent political contestation" (2010, 9) and not as a descriptive category; some of the interdiscipline's most important work involves interrogating its very constitution. For instance, literary critic Ralph E. Rodriguez has argued against deploying *Latinx* "as a taxonomical and aesthetic category" (2018, 3) in cultural criticism, noting that even if such labels are "operational in social and political arenas, that does not mean they have an aesthetic force" (12). Although mindful of these warnings, I have nonetheless used *Latinx* throughout this book because of the force that the term continues to hold in the field of public health. For me, using *Latinx* to denote a population often described in medical literature as "Hispanic" offers a way to bring into conversation cultural workers engaging with health care politics, as well as a means of negotiating between the function of the ethnic label to homogenize, categorize, and pathologize (on one hand) and the artistic and activist projects offering possibilities for redefinition, critique, coalition, and solidarity (on another).

The possibility of coalition and solidarity also means being accountable to the debts that Latinx studies owes to other ethnic studies fields. In this introduction, I have already noted the pivotal role of Black disability scholars in creating the theoretical infrastructure for the body of knowledge now described as crip-of-color critique. Like disability studies, Latinx studies owes a profound debt to Black studies, a debt to which Puerto Rican performance studies scholar Sandra Ruiz eloquently alludes when she reminds us "what Blackness unearths about life and death that other analytics might not ever understand about existence" (2019, 17). As I was researching the chapters that follow, the work of Black studies scholars on HIV/AIDS (Chris Bell), diabetes and metabolic disorders (Richard M. Mizelle Jr., Anthony Ryan Hatch), racialized gender violence (Beth E. Richie), and madness (La Marr Jurelle Bruce, Therí A. Pickens) has been essential for my thinking. In addition, scholars of Asian American studies (Nayan Shah, James Kyung-Jin Lee) have illuminated the discursive links among race, citizenship, migration, and ideologies of health. Ultimately, I find that health functions as what Molina (2014) calls a *racial script*—a racializing narrative that is enacted both in institutional settings and in mundane, everyday interactions; that draws its force from the way it connects to cultural representations and practices used to racialize different groups in different historical periods; and that is available for racialized groups to seize and repurpose (what Molina calls "counterscripting"). In other words, because health works as a racial script, racial health disparities experienced by Latinx people need not be exclusively identifiable as "Latinx concerns" nor be experienced in the same way by *all* Latinx people (or even racialize all Latinx people in the same way) for their racializing effect to matter.

The COVID-19 crisis in the United States helps to illustrate this point. When the novel coronavirus causing COVID-19 was first identified in the United States, it ushered in a wave of racist attacks on Asian and Asian

American communities that (as of this writing more than two years later) continue to escalate. This, in turn, fueled both a more generalized medical racism that prompted immigration restrictions and a broader anti-immigrant sentiment that also affected some (but not all) Latinx communities. By the late spring of 2020, the US-Mexico border was closed, and immigrants from Mexico and Central America were being specifically blamed for COVID-19 outbreaks in rural parts of the southern and midwestern United States. Health and Human Services Secretary Alex Azar attributed outbreaks in meatpacking facilities (Cancryn and Barrón-López 2020) to the "home and social" aspects of workers' lives (not their working conditions), while Florida Governor Ron DeSantis described outbreaks in his state as resulting from immigrant agricultural and construction workers "packed in there like sardines" (Reston 2020) on the buses transporting them to their jobs. Azar and DeSantis did not just devalue the lives of the workers responsible for feeding the rest of the country during a period of disruption in the national food supply but drew from and recirculated the racial script blaming the crisis on Asians and Asian Americans to stigmatize Central American and Mexican immigrant communities, thereby normalizing the disproportionate caseloads and death rates in Latinx communities overall. Like the incidents recounted at the beginning of this introduction—which addressed the convergence of debates over immigration and health care policy—these stories about how a public health crisis heightened and fueled the racialization of diverse Latinx communities across the United States illustrate the need for a specific analysis of how diverse Latinx artists have created counterscripts to disrupt the systemic devaluation of the racialized unwell.

Finally—but importantly—there is the question of why I use the word *Latinx*, a term that has not been universally agreed on by all of the artists whose work I examine in this study (nor by the scholars I cite). As a fairly new term, one the Pew Research Center reminds us has yet to be widely adopted (Noe-Bustamante, Mora, and López 2020), *Latinx* has its detractors, some of whom I find more persuasive than others.[16]

For this reason, it is important to me to specify that I do not use *Latinx* prescriptively or exclusively, and when describing artists and characters who use other identity markers (like Chicana or Latino), I use those. However, I am also inspired by the way Claudia Milian invokes the X as a methodological invitation: "What are we doing with the ethical and political uncertainty of X?" (2019, 7). Answering this question fully, of course, requires its own book (which Milian has already written), but in considering how this project might engage it, I am drawn to the words of Roy Pérez:

I really like the "x" signifier as a reclamation of all kinds of erasure. By using the "x" we expose erasure and refuse it at the same time. I'm a nerd, so for me it invokes the X-men, one of our most culturally visible and diverse narratives about xenophobia and fascism. It's also not lost on me that Black slaves, denied literacy and proper names, were compelled to sign "X" on their freedom papers. When we cross something out, the original remains doggedly just underneath. . . . All told, the "x" has a complex transnational history that is much more rich and full of resistance than a simple story of erasure suggests. I think it's great to be enamored with these linguistic possibilities—Spanish-speaking cultures are all about linguistic play and appropriation. That itself is a kind of freedom. (deOnís 2017, 86)

Pérez's invocation of the mutant superheroes the X-men, in particular, links the X to corporeal nonconformity. His invocation of something crossed out but still visible, remaining "doggedly just underneath," reminds me of how ideas about health and race layer on top of each other. Jonathan M. Metzl defines health as "a set of bodily practices whose ideological work is often rendered invisible by the assumption that it is a monolithic, universal good" (2010, 9). I imagine health as an X that leaves that ideological work partially visible, lurking doggedly just underneath. As a disability studies scholar, moreover, I am mindful of the ways in which nonnormative bodies of all kinds often disrupt gender binaries—or, rather, of the ways in which the gender binary and compulsory able-bodiedness are mutually reinforcing. For these reasons, the X feels right for *this* book, written in *this* moment, although I remain open to the evolution of language and to the possibility that it may not be right for everything I write in the future.

Overview

The chapters that follow cohere around close readings of aesthetic representations in order to foreground my argument that Latinx expressive culture can function as a public health intervention. I state this at the outset because, although I hope the pages that follow will be useful to readers from a wide range of disciplinary backgrounds, I also understand that close readings don't always hold the same interest for those who don't share my scholarly training in cultural criticism or literary studies. (I also recognize that readers who share my training may find some of the close readings too brief!) I use this method of close reading because, although I know that most of my readers will be literary and cultural studies scholars, I also want to bring the artists and writers discussed here to the attention of others who share my interest in health justice, disability politics, and collective wellbeing. Because the chapters each examine a health-related theme as it is depicted in multiple texts, they can feel long. For this reason, I invite readers to skim, to bounce between sections, to pick and choose the analyses that most call to them. I have tried to write in such a way that makes this kind of fragmented reading possible—although, of course, I also welcome the reader who reads cover to cover. One of my goals is to see the texts I analyze here used more regularly in medical and public health training, and I hope that both my analyses and mode of organization (offering a series of short, stand-alone close readings instead of an extended analysis of a single text in each chapter) can help make that possible.

The first two chapters of *Radical Health* take a straightforward approach to the questions that guide this book, examining bodily conditions (HIV/AIDS and diabetes) that are overrepresented in conversations about Latinx communities and health. Chapter 1 examines Latinx cultural engagements with HIV/AIDS spanning the past three decades, from the 1990s until now, by Gil Cuadros, Jaime Cortez and Adela Vázquez, and Rafael Campo. Addressing the prevalence of HIV/AIDS in Latinx communities, these authors refute the myth that HIV/AIDS is a past-tense crisis and prompt us to reimagine the relationship between racial justice and health justice. Chapter 2 focuses on the representation of diabetes in the work of Sonia Sotomayor, Tato Laviera, Virginia Grise and Irma Mayorga, and ire'ne lara silva. I demonstrate how each of these artists refutes mainstream narratives about diabetes and represents the diabetic body as a site of love and political resistance.

The final two chapters take up an invitation by McRuer to imagine disability studies "more capaciously as an epistemological field that makes it possible to know about or intervene in any political or cultural issue" (2010, 164). They also move from an analysis of individual health conditions to a concern with public health. In these chapters, I examine how individualist approaches to health impact approaches to intimate partner violence and immigration policy, even though domestic abuse and immigration are rarely understood as health issues. Chapter 3 examines representations of gender-based and domestic violence in the work of Sonia Nazario, Alynda Mariposa Segarra (via their stage name, Hurray for the Riff Raff), Manuel Muñoz, Rigoberto González, and Angie Cruz to suggest alternate understandings of violence that enable more just solutions. Chapter 4 considers the call of public health scholar Viruell-Fuentes for further analysis of "the health implications of immigration policies" (Viruell-Fuentes, Miranda, and Abdulrahim. 2012, 2102). It examines the health effects of contemporary immigration policy by addressing how Latinx writers (including Reyna Grande, Junot Díaz, Javier Zamora, and Karla Cornejo Villavicencio) have depicted the mental health effects of parent–child separations prompted by immigration.

Instead of ending each chapter with a conclusion that neatly ties together each argument, I end with a *remedio*. Here I use the Spanish word, often translated as *remedy* or *cure*, to think not only about the remedies that these texts imagine but also about the stakes of *remediation*, a word that is often used to refer to the reversal of damage but can also mean the translation from one medium to another. What does it mean, I ask throughout this book, to translate questions that are often seen as the purview of health professionals into an aesthetic medium? Why does it matter, in other words, that I have approached these public health concerns not through epidemiological investigation but through cultural criticism? Often my *remedios* take the form of meditating on the intellectual journey that brought me to a particular topic or the unanswered questions about it that continue to linger for me.

This is the especially the case with my final *remedio*, the book's short concluding chapter, in which I describe the personal experiences that brought me to this project. In this final meditation, I make explicit how my own social location—as a white, crip ciswoman who is often assumed (and for a long time assumed myself) to be nondisabled—has shaped my relationship to the texts I analyze and to the ideology of health. It is a common gesture among white scholars like myself who work in ethnic studies to invoke experiences demonstrating allyship, solidarity, and common cause (often filtered through shared social class background, shared neighborhoods, childhood friends, etc.). I believe such gestures are necessary, but I also believe that it is important for us to understand their limits. In this *remedio*, I wanted to tell a harder story, exploring how white supremacy and ableism have shaped the white liberalism in which I was raised—and which led me to both Latinx and disability studies. I have struggled with the question of where to place this story in the book, whether to start or end with it. In the end, I have opted to begin with the texts that have given me the concept of radical health, to center the artists and writers who give me faith that health is a concept worth reexamining, a concept that can be radically reimagined. Yet as I insist throughout this book that radical health can be envisioned from conditions of deep unwellness, I offer in the final chapter an account of my own attempt to do so.

1

Unprotected Texts

Queer Latinx Expression in the Aftermath of AIDS

As I complete this chapter, I am told that a pandemic is ending. After nearly two years of masking and social distancing, people in places with medical resources have been vaccinated against COVID-19 and are joyfully abandoning precautions. My employer expects me to return to teaching in-person classes. Bars, restaurants, and entertainment venues are open and—I hear—serving full-capacity crowds. Airports are full again. Meanwhile, those who are (or who live with people who are) immunosuppressed or ineligible for vaccination obsessively scour the news for updates on new coronavirus variants, don masks, and avoid public gatherings.

I started writing this chapter years before the COVID-19 pandemic. What first inspired it was my love for Gil Cuadros's 1994 mixed-genre collection *City of God*, which explores living with HIV/AIDS in the late 1980s and early 1990s. Many things have changed since Cuadros wrote the poems and prose pieces in that gorgeous volume, notably the development in 1996 of highly active antiretroviral therapy (HAART), which has transformed the experience of living with the virus for those who can access it, whose lives accommodate its rigid requirements, and who tolerate its side effects. The publication of Cuadros's book aligns it temporally with what might now be called a canon of HIV/AIDS writing, although at the time I came to read it as a graduate student in the mid-2000s, it felt to me that hardly anyone was working on or even thinking about Cuadros, that his work was treated as a document of an earlier time. But the book would not let me go, and ten years after reading it for the first time, I began writing in earnest about *City of God*—and also asking myself what HIV/AIDS literary criticism in the HAART era might look like. I was driven by a belief in the continued relevance of *City of God* even as it chronicles an earlier moment in the HIV/AIDS pandemic. Indeed, despite a general sense in the United States that medical advances enable us to speak of HIV/AIDS in the past, the virus remains an urgent concern for many, particularly those belonging to communities for which treating and preventing HIV/AIDS is not considered profitable. Teaching aesthetic representations of HIV/AIDS, especially the work of Cuadros, to students in Texas—a state where abstinence-only education remains common in K–12 schools—I have found myself routinely asked to explain basic facts about how HIV is transmitted. Many of my students, denied access to life-sustaining information about the virus, belong to groups vulnerable to infection: they are often young, economically disenfranchised, queer and gender-nonconforming, and/or Latinx. Although I do not conflate the social conditions in which Cuadros wrote *City of God* with those my students and I navigate, I recognize that the same cultural forces he chronicles and critiques—white supremacy, heteropatriarchy, disease stigma—shape the world in which I teach his work today, giving his words continued urgency every time I read them.

I also do not conflate the COVID-19 pandemic, which approaches its second year as I write my own words, with the HIV/AIDS pandemic. If anything, it was HIV/AIDS art and activism that shaped my experience of COVID-19, not my experience of COVID-19 that shaped my interpretation of the texts I discuss in this chapter. The texts examined here have taught me that cultural representations of illness reveal who is valued in a society and who is not. In particular, they demonstrate that social narratives locating an ongoing public health crisis in the past tense effectively work to construct the people still affected by that crisis as unimportant, lacking value, expendable. In the case of both HIV/AIDS and COVID-19, medical solutions became available, but biomedicine did not address the cultural devaluation of those most affected. And in both cases those with access to care declared the pandemic over while those without continued to die. As Jih-Fei Cheng, Alexandra Juhasz, and Nishant Shahani write of HIV/AIDS, the crisis did not end; rather, "its effects became scattered among populations whose proximity to death is naturalized as inevitable or axiomatic, or whose access to representation or representability allows their crises to go unrecognized" (2020, 4). Although comparisons between HIV/AIDS and COVID-19 only go so far, it is instructive to think about them together because, as Karma R. Chávez has noted, both reveal "the deep logic of white supremacist, anti-Black, settler colonial nation-states like the United States" (2021, vii). It is this logic that the texts examined here—all of which I read from a post-HAART vantage point—disrupt.

This chapter examines the work of artists and activists—Gil Cuadros, Jaime Cortez, Adela Vázquez, and Rafael Campo—for whom the ongoing prevalence of HIV/AIDS in Latinx communities demands an ethic of radical health. As elaborated in the introduction, I use the phrase *radical health* to describe a relationship to health that emerges when people whose health status subjects them to stigma and racialization simultaneously reject the devaluation of their bodyminds and advocate for access to resources that support wellbeing (including, but not limited to, health care). I examine texts from three decades of Latinx HIV/AIDS art: Cuadros's 1994 mixed-genre book *City of God*; Cortez's 2004 graphic biography, *Sexile*, depicting the life of trans activist Vázquez; and Campo's 2013 poetry collection *Alternative Medicine*. Engaging with these artists in the fourth decade of the HIV/AIDS pandemic provides powerful insights for resisting the logics that present HIV/AIDS as belonging elsewhere (in a distant past or on another continent), that treat the bodies and lives of those affected as disposable, and that pathologize sexual risk-taking while failing to address structural inequities.

My title for this chapter, "Unprotected Texts," is a nod to Cuadros (who titled one of his most arresting prose pieces "Unprotected") and captures his trenchant critique of how queer Latinx people have been systemically unprotected from HIV/AIDS, a critique shared by Cortez, Vázquez, and Campo. The term *unprotected* designates both a category of socially unsanctioned sexual acts (those undertaken without efforts to avoid contagion) and a state of what Lisa Marie Cacho calls "racialized rightlessness." For Cacho, the "unprotected" include "the deviant, the non-American, the nonnormative, the pathologized, and the recalcitrant—the legally repudiated 'others' of human value in the United States" (2012, 18). I argue that for queer and racialized people living with HIV/AIDS, these two meanings are not so distinct. With mainstream recognition of (some) gay rights activism, the stigma once attached to queer sex now adheres to sex deemed "unsafe," "risky," or "unprotected." Despite liberal/progressive displays of "tolerance" for queer identities, denunciation and even criminalization of "unprotected" sex continues, constructing those who participate in it as deserving everything from disease to prosecution.[1] As Carlos Ulises Decena (2008, 399) argues, a "regime of compulsory disclosure" now regulates sexual citizenship. Given the number of states with criminal statutes against seropositive sex regardless of precautionary measures, for some HIV-positive individuals, *all* sex is legally "unprotected."[2] Reading *City of God, Sexile,* and *Alternative Medicine* in the purported aftermath of HIV/AIDS prompts scrutiny of who can access the protection of socially legitimated sexuality and who is left unprotected.

Not only do Cuadros, Cortez, Vázquez, and Campo offer perspectives informed by different relationships to HIV/AIDS—that of a person living with AIDS, that of HIV/AIDS activists, and that of a physician—the publication dates of the texts discussed here span two crucial decades in the history of both the virus and the US health care system: 1994–2013. As noted, the earliest of these texts (*City of God*) predates a medical triumph (HAART) by just two years; however, its publication also coincides with political disappointments and losses. These include the collapse of President Bill Clinton's effort to create a national health care plan and the decline of direct-action anti-AIDS activism by groups like ACT UP (the AIDS Coalition to Unleash Power), whose local chapters across the United States dissolved throughout the mid-to-late 1990s. The most recent of these texts (Campo's *Alternative Medicine*) was published in 2013, between the passage of the 2010 Patient Protection and Affordable Care Act (ACA) and its full implementation in 2014; this text also precedes by just three years the rise to power of Donald Trump, whose presidential campaign was fueled by promises to repeal the ACA. The period addressed in this chapter, then, is one of intense public negotiation about who deserves health and who does not. Sociologist Deborah B. Gould describes the history of HIV/AIDS in the United States as the story "of a government of a wealthy, ostensibly democratic country unmoved by the deaths of hundreds, thousands, and finally hundreds of thousands of its own inhabitants, largely because the overwhelming majority of them were gay and bisexual men, and the others were seen as similarly expendable: drug users as well as poor men and women, a disproportionate number of whom were black and Latino/a" (2009, 45). As I write, the violent apathy Gould critiques continues even as its target has expanded and proliferated (from the person with AIDS to the "essential worker" whose job in childcare, delivery, meatpacking, or other low-wage sectors places them at high risk of exposure to COVID-19).

In a society that continues to practice such callousness, Cuadros, Cortez, Vázquez, and Campo offer a powerful ethic of radical health.

Gil Cuadros's AZTlán

Cuadros began writing after testing positive for HIV in 1987, while in his early twenties; he died of AIDS-related causes in 1996 at age thirty-four.[3] His only book is *City of God*, a collection of autobiographical short prose and poetry whose status in Chicanx and gay literary canons is ambivalent. Although *City of God* is often footnoted as an essential gay Chicanx text, there was for many years surprisingly little scholarship on it.[4] The years of very sparse critical engagement likely result from the book's uneasy fit with celebratory impulses that have proven remarkably persistent in both Chicanx and queer studies. Cuadros's frank depictions of power imbalances between young Chicanos and their older white lovers can be distressing to read, and even friendly readers, like reviewer Jesse Monteagudo, note that his words "quiver with despair" (1995, 34). By contrast, Heather Love observes an enduring "need to resist damage and to affirm queer existence" in queer studies (2007, 3); Leticia Alvarado similarly notes the emphasis on positive emotions like "pride over shame, bravery over fear" (2018, 2) in the representations prioritized in Latinx social justice organizing. When the histories of Latinx and queer activism are told in ways that insist on affirmation and pride, stories like those told by Cuadros—of loss, ambivalence, and trauma—become more difficult to tell.

While many critics have emphasized the alienation of Cuadros and his characters—both from their Chicanx families and from predominantly white gay communities—I argue that *City of God* offers a vision of radical health and sexual access in a hostile social environment. Simply put, I find Cuadros foregrounding the complexities of his location *within* Mexican and gay Los Angeles, not his isolation from them. Challenging health care inequities and interrogating conceptions of "healthy" sexuality, *City of God* retains its urgency at a time when comprehensive health care access and information for young Latinx queers remains tenuous. In particular, in the prose pieces "My Aztlan: White Place" and "Unprotected" and in the poem "There Are Places You Don't Walk at Night, Alone," Cuadros incisively foregrounds the consequences of a societal failure to treat sexual health as a matter of collective concern.

"My Aztlan: White Place," Cuadros's best-known text, is a prose piece offering an autobiographical account of his fraught relationships with his parents and white lover.[5] Of all the pieces in the collection, "My Aztlan" most directly engages with prominent themes of Chicanx literature, including Aztlán and the Los Angeles freeway system.[6] With a reference to AZT (azidothymidine), the first antiretroviral drug approved by the US government for the treatment of HIV/AIDS, the piece also depicts an important moment in the medical history of the virus. The body of the text's protagonist links Chicanx and HIV/AIDS histories as it registers his profound ambivalence toward both the biomedical promise of drug therapy (then less effective and more encumbered by side effects) and the political promise of Aztlán. "My Aztlan" is a first-person monologue that begins with its narrator "stinking drunk, driving down the wrong freeway" (Cuadros 1994, 52) after a night in the West Hollywood bars; he calls his mother from a freeway callbox before returning to his apartment, where he vomits, showers, and masturbates. The freeway connects the narrator's (mostly white) gay milieu to his family. For instance, the narrator asks himself why he is attracted to "those West Hollywood bar types—blond hair, blue eyes" (53) before revealing that the "wrong freeway" on which he is driving has displaced his childhood home: "I was born below this freeway, in a house with a picket fence now plowed under" (54). His drunk driving between West Hollywood and his former home further emphasizes this risky back-and-forth between communities.

The narrator's tenuous position in his family becomes clear as he locates an explicit description of sex in his parents' bed. This occurs not because he himself has sex in that bed but because his mother lies awake in it, imagining her son: "She doesn't want to think about the white man who infected me. 'He might as well have shot you,' she said once. My mother let me know that she turns in her sleep, sick at the thought of his dick up my ass or in my mouth. A milky white fluid floats in my body's space, breaks into the secret bonding of her sex, my father's sex, and the marriage of their cells" (54). Passages like this have led critics to read this narrator as isolated from his family. For instance, Rafael Pérez-Torres asserts that the narrator's sexuality "breaks the family bonds between husband and wife, mother and son" (2006, 165). However, I emphasize that the narrator uses the phrase "breaks *into*" instead of the word "breaks," evoking not rupture but brutal comingling. Ernesto Javier Martínez's observation that "queer experiences are actually *coproduced and shared* by larger collectives, even though these larger collectives often deny their own implicatedness in queer sociality" (2013, 113) informs my interpretation: the mother's sickness at her son's sexuality results from her awareness that her own sexuality, like that of her son, resists containment within the normative heteropatriarchal family. Further evidence that it is *shared* desires, experiences, and practices that cause the mother's disgust emerges when the narrator recalls his father coming home drunk to forcefully snuggle and tickle him. He states that "my mother hated my father like this" (55–56) and that "my lover never understood why I hated to be tickled, why I liked to be tied up" (56), alluding to unspoken understandings between mother and son due to the ways in which both have experienced the father's pugnacious affections.[7]

The narrator's fraught position in his family parallels his relationships to both Chicano nationalism and biomedical treatment, prompting the story's arresting title identifying Aztlán as a "white place." He imagines his childhood home "still intact, buried under dirt and asphalt, dust and neglect," and defines this home as "my Aztlan," but reveals that it is not a safe space: "All it takes is a well-chosen phrase to cave in: Mom, why did you burn my hands with the iron and say it was an accident? tattoo my arms with the car's cigarette lighter? make me wish your wish, that I was never born?" (55). This is not the utopic Aztlán of nationalist yearnings. Pérez-Torres (2006, 165) astutely notes that the first three letters of the word *Aztlán* are AZT, an observation I find suggestive because the story's reference to AZT involves vomiting: "I run to the toilet to puke, a steady stream pours out of my mouth. An empty AZT shell comes, then foam. It floats on the water's tension, circles the bowl and disappears. It has become ritual to lie on the cold tile, stare at the mold patched ceiling, skip another set of pills, what some people call hope" (Cuadros 1994, 56). A common side effect of AZT thus becomes a metaphor for the narrator's relationship to political communities, as his physical rejection of the "hope" of AZT parallels his ambivalence toward the "hope" of Aztlán. Vomiting the AZT shell represents a denunciation of cultural logics that treat HIV/AIDS solely as a medical problem rather than also as a call for social change, while the revelation of his Aztlán's painful history similarly denounces the nationalist ideal that ethnic self-determination alone can resolve legacies of heteropatriarchy and white supremacy. Although Cuadros could not have foreseen AZT's current importance for HIV/AIDS therapy, he recognized that its availability would not end the political exclusion of queer men of color with HIV/AIDS.[8] Now that, as Juana María Rodríguez argues, "HIV infection and AIDS have become manageable conditions for those who can manage, where managing is often a code for being white, educated, employed, and connected to the dominant gay male scene" (2020, 280–81), Cuadros's critique of this exclusion is as urgent as ever. Today, HIV-positive individuals will live longer if they can access the right medications, but traces of the same sociopolitical exclusions that Cuadros illuminates linger in debates over health care access, the criminalization of seropositive sex, and the narrative that HIV/AIDS is no longer a crisis.

The text's final lines depict the narrator imagining himself simultaneously buried in his family home and becoming the freeway that has destroyed it: "I can feel my body becoming tar, limbs divide, north and south. My house smells of earth and it rumbles from the traffic above. White clay sifts through the ceiling. My bones shine in the dark" (58). For the reader aware of the Chicana lesbian literary tradition that precedes Cuadros's writing, this image of his narrator's body as a freeway poignantly evokes the title of the collection *This Bridge Called My Back*, edited by Cherríe Moraga and Gloria Anzaldúa (1983), which similarly critiqued the systemic exclusion of the multiply marginalized. Bridges and freeways provide necessary connections, but both are transitory; as permanent homes, they are untenable.

"Unprotected"

"Unprotected" depicts a sexual encounter between two men who meet at a West Los Angeles bar, one HIV-positive (the narrator, who shares biographical details with Cuadros) and one who claims to be HIV-negative. The story begins the day after, with the seropositive man preoccupied by the odor of hand lotion: "It is faint in my beard. It is underneath my nails and I can smell it when I bring food to my mouth. It is here in my bed. It smells of cock and ass. It smells unnatural. It smells unsafe" (59). The scent represents his ambivalence about the previous night: he was drunk at a bar when a man invited him to his condo; he revealed his serostatus to the man, who then initiated sex; afterward, he caught a bus home. Although the narrator uses the adjectives "unnatural" and "unsafe" to describe lingering sexual odors, he never specifies whether any precautions were used, thus inviting the reader to reevaluate what it means to be un/protected in *any* sexual encounter—especially when accounting not only for serodiscordance but also for race and class differences.

"Unprotected" is a powerful indictment of what disability scholar Abby Wilkerson calls "economies of sexual gratitude, in which sexual partners . . .

whose bodies are further from cultural norms of health, fitness, or attractiveness, are expected or assumed to feel grateful to partners . . . considered attractive or fit by conventional standards" (2012, 198). Although narrated in the first person by the seropositive man, "Unprotected" contains few statements of his desires, only descriptions of his actions: "I staggered out of the bar, following a man whose name I didn't hear" (61–62). The narrator is surprised by the man's attention: "I didn't think I was attractive enough, especially now with the virus" (62). When the man initiates sex, the narrator tells himself: "Shut up, you're going to die anyway. Enjoy this because this is going to be your last time . . . I knew I would let him fuck me, there wasn't even an afterthought" (69). The evacuation from the story of the HIV-positive man's desires, even as Cuadros's use of the first person seems to give this character narrative control, illustrates what Chris Bell has called a disregard for the "oft-maligned and rarely discussed wishes of HIV-positive individuals" in mainstream representations (2012, 226).

The neglect for the concerns of HIV-positive people that Bell critiques is particularly evident in rhetoric around so-called bug chasing, in which HIV-negative people seek out HIV-positive sex partners.[9] As Tim Dean notes, the cultural visibility of bug chasing (and, more generally, the emergence of bareback subcultures) is linked to the availability of antiretroviral therapy (and hence the possibility of being HIV-positive without developing AIDS); he cautions that the practice cannot be understood without "acknowledging how, partly in reaction to the excessive pathologizing of persons with AIDS, the pathogen has been reinterpreted as desirable" (2009, 54). "Unprotected" predates the conditions Dean describes and never employs the term *bug chasing*, but the text hints that the man is specifically seeking out an HIV-positive partner. After both men reveal their serostatus, the following conversation takes place:

> He sat back in his chair, lighting a cigarette. "Do you feel comfortable with this?"
>
> I said, "I feel a little weird."
>
> "Like how?"
>
> "Like I'm infectious material." He winced at the remark. I saw myself being transported in an orange-red garbage bag, getting tossed out by sallow-colored gloves.
>
> Recomposed, he said rather smugly, almost challenging me, "Well, if you don't feel right about this, it's fine with me. I accept myself for what I am." I thought it must be easy when you're negative. (66)

This dialogue reveals the complexity of serodiscordant sexual encounters, given both the stigmas surrounding HIV/AIDS and the prevalence of laws criminalizing HIV transmission. Dean observes that when men make "the virus central to their erotic lives," they "have sex not only with other men but also with a virus" (2009, 17). Telling his sexual partner that he feels "like infectious material," the narrator shows how being interpellated as a pathogen can be a hostile experience, even among those who purport to oppose the pathologization of people with AIDS.[10]

"Unprotected" offers several clues that the sex it depicts is dishonestly negotiated. The first comes before the men arrive at the condo, when the man pressures the narrator to consume more alcohol and makes casual references to HIV/AIDS victim-blaming: "We stopped at Rocky's liquor . . . I asked for a Pepsi. He came back with Coronas and a pot of spider mums. . . . [H]e told me they were for a friend who was sick in the hospital. He started talking about his condo, saying it was real nice. He then told me he had brought someone up there once and was ripped off. He talked philosophically of Louise Hay" (63).[11] Arriving at the man's "beautiful" (63) and "immaculate" (64) condo does not reassure the narrator, especially after the man states that he is HIV-negative: "I felt or thought that maybe he was positive. He talked about his sick friend, the Hay group, it seemed probable that he had the virus" (65). The narrator describes himself as "limp and unexcited" (68) before describing the sex itself: "I thought . . . that if I could get his leg off me, I could get up and put my clothes back on and leave. . . . My wrists were held down by the weight of his hands and body" (68). Afterward, although the man invites him to spend the night, he cannot sleep. In these ways, the story places under scrutiny the cultural logic that would construct HIV-positive people as a sexual threat (a cultural logic that has led to HIV-specific criminal statutes), revealing how HIV-positive individuals are at sexual risk.

While texts like "Unprotected" depict their narrators' social vulnerability, prompting critics like Raúl Homero Villa to see Cuadros's characters as "doubly displaced" (2000, 141) from Mexican and gay communities, I posit that this vulnerability highlights the efforts to forge a sense of belonging in hostile spaces. Here I emphasize the story's conclusion:

I ran to catch the bus and it waited for me. It was filled with Mexicanos, some from South America. The men all looked at me as I entered, and I took my seat quickly. I was afraid they could smell the shit that was in my beard, see the sticky shine of cum over my body, and know what I had done that night. Each one of those short, stocky men with their black hair and Indian features would know. The seat next to me was empty until a young Mexican man sat down. He spread his legs open till they touched mine. The bus tore down the street, hitting a pothole. It jarred the riders and made my neighbor rub his leg against mine. He smiled at me. I pulled my legs together, closing them tight. I fell asleep against the window that was cracked open, my hands acting as a pillow, breathing in the exhaust from outside and the lotion that was over my hands, heavy as spring air. (69–70)

Paul Allatson's analysis of this passage aligns with Villa's reading: "In this Latinized space, Cuadros is fearful that his night's sexual acts will somehow stigmatize him" and attempts "to limit the signifying import of his body so that he will appear neither Chicano nor queer" (2007, 36). There is limited evidence for this argument; for instance, the narrator is "afraid" that the men will "know what I had done." Nonetheless, there is also evidence that although the narrator is not fully at ease on the bus, he is *more* at ease here than anywhere else. First, he knows how and where to catch the bus and perceives it to wait for him.[12] Second, unlike in the condo, the narrator is able to sleep.

Given these details, the narrator's concern about the men on the bus "knowing" him deserves closer scrutiny. Unlike the men on the bus, this character's parents refuse to know him: "They worried about my ARC diagnosis, but they would never ask about it" (59). Furthermore, the narrator resents that the man in the condo brags about living with "nothing to hide" (64), even refusing to cover his windows, while he has to "hide everything" (64), from the "gold wedding band that is on a chain my parents had given me" to "the blue-red pinpoints on my veins, a sign of bimonthly blood workups and the virus" (64). These details suggest that feeling known by the men on the bus has a more positive valence than Allatson acknowledges, even as it is undeniably tinged with trepidation, for despite his fear of judgment the narrator experiences a mutual recognition with these men that he experiences with few others. Among these working-class Latinx men, he feels what might be called a nascent sense of belonging, one that does not mitigate the violence of the previous night (the odor of the lotion lingers) but that also does not threaten him. Here we might look more closely at the man who sits next to him, rubs legs with him, and smiles. I read this as a sexual advance, and I find it significant that the narrator rebuffs it but is still able to sleep after being unable to do so at the condo. Disrupting the economy of sexual gratitude, the narrator's refusal to acquiesce produces a sense of ease that, while not total or perfect, permits a moment of rest.[13]

This ambiguous ending might seem to bolster criticism of the political vision of *City of God*. Pérez-Torres, for instance, sees Cuadros offering "emotional, spiritual, and physical transformations at the expense of social change or queer political agency" (2006, 192–93). I posit instead that the impulse to read Cuadros's characters as lacking political agency corresponds to a resistance/victim binary in which, as Antonio Viego notes, "gay Chicano and Latino men are often figured as the weak links in political movements for Chicana/o, Latina/o ethnic, racial empowerment" (1999, 120). More than offering a concrete vision of what social change or queer political agency might look like, Cuadros reveals the difficulty of imagining either when, as Cacho reminds us, "the very personhood of unprotected residents in this nation is formalized in law as irrelevant" (2012, 24). We might instead read Cuadros's depictions of seropositive Chicano gay men inhabiting spaces like the bus as a search for belonging.

Reading the bus as a site of potential belonging, if not a fully realized political community, requires considering the kind of belonging that a bus might represent. A bus is in motion, migratory, porous, permeable, accessible to people whose economic resources prevent them from purchasing cars or whose disabilities prevent them from driving; it is a site at which heterogeneous people continually board and depart, mingling like bodily fluids. A bus is publicly funded and maintained, often a refuge for people experiencing homelessness, and a site of unexpected connections. At the same time, a bus can also be unsafe, as public transportation is often associated with harassment, theft, assault, and other petty crimes; to ride the bus regularly is to come into contact with rude, offensive, threatening, and sometimes violent people. As a mode of travel, a bus is indirect, slow, inconvenient, bumpy, and uncomfortable. Concluding on a bus, "Unprotected" offers a vision of what we might call an unprotected political community, one that is radically inclusive and open but not always safe or easy to inhabit.

"There Are Places You Don't Walk at Night, Alone"

"There Are Places You Don't Walk at Night, Alone" is set in two East Los Angeles neighborhoods, Boyle Heights and Silver Lake, and depicts attachments of its speaker to other men of color, further exploring the vision of community that surfaces at the end of "Unprotected." The poem consists of three episodes that read like numbered chapters. Each begins with a list of streets and describes a violent encounter on or around them. The streets in the first and third episode are located in Boyle Heights, a neighborhood that was predominantly Mexican and Chicanx in the 1990s, whereas those in the second are near the gay bar The Detour (now the 4100 Bar and no longer a gay establishment) in Silver Lake, a historically working-class area with a large Latinx population and an extensive queer history.[14] The movement between these neighborhoods illustrates the speaker's presence in multiple communities, but the poem gives twice the narrative space to Boyle Heights that it gives to Silver Lake. Furthermore, the most violent encounter takes place inside Detour, challenging Allatson's suggestion that the poem is mostly about "homophobic violence perpetrated by cholos in East Los Angeles barrios" (2007, 35). Finally, by starting in Boyle Heights and returning at the end, the poem claims space for its speaker in a Mexican community. This belonging is represented by bandannas; each episode features bandannas of different colors that signal community ties.

The Boyle Heights streets in the poem's first episode are featured so frequently in Chicanx art as to be iconic: "Whittier Blvd, Beverly, Atlantic,/ over by Johnson's Market,/or the projects on Brooklyn" (Cuadros 1994, 112).[15] This episode invokes a childhood memory from a time when

> There weren't any Bloods
> or Crips yet on TV and everyone
> bought bandannas
> at Sav-On. Combinations
> of blue and red packages,
> the cellophane crinkled in the hand. (112)

Although these lines appear to invoke a time before widespread social panic over gang violence, the speaker reveals that the neighborhood has always been violent for him: "They'd cuff me from behind,/their hands lingering on my neck, saying/'Come here, faggot, kiss me'" (112). This poem also shows homophobia coexisting with queer recognition and violation, describing the hands of the *cholos* "lingering" on the speaker's neck as they demand kisses. It ends with the speaker being kicked by the *cholos*, revealing its politics of brotherhood to exist only as a possibility, but its disconcertingly gentle language—the *cholos*' "warm and brown" (112) eyes and "leather soles/that brushed the hair out of my face" (112)—suggests a speaker who feels both violent exclusion and uneasy belonging in his neighborhood.

The poem's second episode is its most violent; it begins with a list of streets clustered around The Detour and describes the speaker's lover being stabbed and then denied treatment:

Marc's t-shirt turned red,
the paramedics wouldn't touch him.
I filled in the holes,
my fingers adding pressure
on a hunter-green bandanna. (113)

Before the incident, the speaker instructs his lover how to enter the bar: "I told him you had to walk/with an attitude" (113), suggesting that his up-bringing in Boyle Heights has prepared him for the violence at The Detour (and, therefore, that the two spaces are not as oppositional as some Cuadros criticism suggests). Second, although the attacker who stabs Marc is not identified, the bar's location suggests that the aggressor is likely *not* one of the cholos from the previous episode. Finally, unlike in the other two episodes, the violence is not only individual but also structural, perpetrated by the attacker as well as by paramedics willing to let Marc bleed to death. This episode, then, continues the critique of biomedical responses to HIV/AIDS in "My Aztlan" through its reminder that homophobic violence is also enacted through medical neglect. It is important to note, as well, that although advances in knowledge about HIV prevention have reduced the occurrence of overt medical malpractice like that described here, debates over who deserves medical care continue, with life-or-death consequences for those who are poor, racialized, and/or immunosuppressed.

The poem's final episode returns to Boyle Heights, where the speaker waits for a bus with the cholos from the first episode and notices them watching gay men enter a nearby adult bookstore, "the pink bandannas folded like/their own blue" (114). Here the bus is again a site of queer recognition, hinted at in the first episode and now rendered more explicit by the parallel between the bandannas. At the same time, the narrator imagines himself as a perpetrator of the same violence enacted on him during his youth:

I want to smash them into the windows,
make them spread their legs,
my boots kicking them wide,
let my spit drip
into their ears,
seep into their brains,
tell them how much I love them. (114)

Although the final line of this poem positions the cholos as objects of queer desire, it even more radically signals the speaker's desire for a communal identification that includes queerness. The embrace described in this poem is informed by a long history of sexualized violence that cannot be put aside. The poem's hope—and *City of God*'s overall vision of radical health—lies not in the fulfillment of the speaker's desire for belonging but in the persistence of that desire in the face of violence.[16]

Sexile: Radical Prevention

Although a core argument of *Radical Health* is that expressive culture can function as a health intervention, the 2004 graphic biography *Sexile*, a collaboration between the Chicano artist Jaime Cortez and the Cuban American transgender activist Adela Vázquez, is the only text I examine in this book that was specifically created for this purpose. Yet although *Sexile* was published and distributed in partnership with two HIV/AIDS service organizations, it doesn't immediately present as an HIV prevention text.[17] It contains no discussion of T cells, no demonstrations of effective condom use, no warnings about intravenous needles. For readers unaware of its origin, *Sexile* presents simply as a graphic narrative. Illustrated by Cortez, *Sexile* recounts the life of Vázquez: her childhood and early adulthood in revolutionary Cuba; her relocation to the United States during the Mariel boatlift; her time in a resettlement camp in Fort Chaffee, Arkansas; her life in Los Angeles; her gender correction process; and her strategies for survival. In the entire sixty-six-page book, only four pages refer to HIV/AIDS, and in many cases they do so indirectly: three describe how Adela starts using condoms after getting her first sexually transmitted disease in 1981; and one notes that when employed as a sex worker she refused clients offering to pay extra for sex without condoms. By comparison, the entire second chapter of *Sexile*—a total of eight pages, twice the space devoted to HIV/AIDS—is dedicated to the Mariel boatlift (which enabled Vázquez to leave Cuba). *Sexile* thus prompts the question: What does the history of Cuban migration to the United States have to do with HIV prevention?

Both Cortez and Patrick "Pato" Hebert (of AIDS Project Los Angeles, one of *Sexile*'s nonprofit sponsors) begin to answer this question in the prefatory notes to *Sexile*. In the foreword, Hebert writes: "HIV prevention is too often preoccupied with tiny pieces of what we do rather than the fullness of what we feel and the vastness of who we are becoming. *Sexile* is special because it reminds us of the power of storytelling, laughter, honesty, mistakes, magic and perseverance" (2004, v). Cortez, for his part, states the need for "an HIV prevention publication centered on the life of an unapologetic wildchild with a highly developed taste for sex, adventure and controlled substances" and notes "that Adela's life is extraordinarily rich in lessons on being resilient and negotiating risk" (2004, vii). Perhaps most revealing is Cortez's note in the acknowledgments identifying the text as the "new baby" of the "diasporic folk of the Proyecto Village." This is a reference to the AIDS service organization Proyecto ContraSIDA por Vida ("Proyecto"), active in San Francisco's Mission District from 1993 to 2005, whose approach to HIV prevention offers a model for radical health interventions. While no reference to Proyecto appears in the text itself, Hebert, Cortez, and Vázquez (along with a number of prominent Bay Area Latinx artists, activists, and academics) have all had Proyecto affiliations; Vázquez was a longtime staff member, serving as outreach coordinator. Juana María Rodríguez (another Proyecto comrade) describes Proyecto as distinguished by "its commitment to multi-gender organizing, its declared posture of providing sex-positive programming, and its commitment to harm reduction as a model for prevention and treatment" (2003, 49). These elements, visible throughout *Sexile*, align with the theory of radical health I advance in this book.

Like the work of Proyecto—sex-positive but also deeply engaged with the effects of shame, alienation, repression, disenfranchisement, white supremacy, and colonialism—*Sexile* moves between emotional registers, presenting Adela's life in ways that are both celebratory and painful. "Remember disgrace?" Adela asks in the opening chapter. "Back then in country-ass Cuba, everybody knew it was a disgrace to have a baby but no husband. Soon as I came out my mama's pussy, my grandma and grandpa, they adopted me and brought me to live with them on the family orange farm. My grandma, my tías, they loved my bastard ass. My childhood was so beautiful, but I can't say too much about it . . . because it hurts to remember" (5). This passage—accompanied by images of a house with a tiled roof set among orange trees, a glamorous woman seated on a couch, and a masculine child in a fishing boat with an older man (presumably Adela and her grandfather)—alludes to sexual repression, upends the expected script of a trans child experiencing familial rejection, and invokes the pain of exile. Asserting all at once that a trans child can cultivate beautiful memories in a place that treats sex as a "disgrace" and that the pain of separation from "country-ass Cuba" lingers after exile, *Sexile* engages in what Alberto Sandoval-Sánchez has called a *politics of abjection,* a concept that serves as a traveling companion to my own formulation of radical health.[18] Sandoval-Sánchez writes:

The politics of abjection that I suggest is rooted in Latino queer bodies with AIDS—*unos cuerpos* marked by race, ethnicity, class, sexuality, AIDS, and migration, *unos cuerpos* that endanger and trouble the cohesion of the social order by destabilizing the borders between normal and deviant, insider and outsider, sameness and difference, health and illness, life and death. . . . [T]o embrace abjection is to undo, in some part, racism, shame, homophobia, and the fear of death, allowing for a source of self-empowerment and a liberating counterhegemonic force of bodies in revolt. (2005, 548)

Of the boundaries that Sandoval-Sánchez identifies, those separating health/illness and life/death are of particular interest to me, as they tend to be reified in mainstream health interventions. Such work is dominated by "expert" voices, aligned with health/life and distinguished from the "at-risk" subject who receives the information and is implicitly aligned with illness/death.

To elaborate the significance of *Sexile*'s dissolution of these binaries, I return to the question with which I began this section: *What does the Mariel boatlift have to do with HIV prevention?* Between April and October 1980, more than 125,000 Cubans left their country through Mariel Harbor after a man drove a truck into the Peruvian embassy and approximately ten thousand people took refuge there seeking to leave the country. As Susana Peña describes it:

The Mariel boatlift was an immigration crisis and a public relations nightmare for both the United States and Cuba. As images of thousands of Cubans wanting to leave Cuba circulated in the international media, Castro began a disparagement campaign in which he labeled the migrants *escoria*, lumpen proletariat, *antisociales*, prostitutes, and homosexuals. . . . For U.S. president Jimmy Carter, this apparently uncontrollable migration of undesirables (during an election year) was far from ideal. To make matters worse, the Cuban government's insults were echoed among Miami's existing Cuban American population as they began noticing that the Mariel migrants were more likely to be black, poor, and less educated than previous Cuban immigrants. (2013, x)

For Peña and others, a key component of the Mariel stigma had to do with the large number of queer migrants who left Cuba during the crisis; she documents how both "the Cuban and U.S. states stigmatized, identified, and tracked the movement of sexually transgressive bodies within and across their national borders" (2013, xiii). *Sexile* makes visible the material effects of this stigma; Adela notes: "Some people in Cuba say that the day the Marielitos left was the day Cuba flushed the toilet. I say flush away, bitch" (21). This pronouncement is followed four pages later with a series of images of Adela, trying to get to Mariel, beaten by an angry mob incited by Castro's disparagement campaign.[19] Throughout the sections depicting her departure from Cuba and arrival in a resettlement camp, Adela is shown with a black eye and bloodstained shirt, markers of this brutal beating. While ostensibly she is targeted for her lack of patriotism, it is clear that the violence is also directed at her queer body.

Although Adela's migration brings her new economic and political freedoms, ultimately culminating in her decision to undergo gender-affirming medical procedures, it is not narrated as a straightforward journey from repression to liberation.[20] Adela has many lovers in Cuba: "Yes, mama had plenty, thank you very much" (9). Even her time in the resettlement camp is memorable for the fact that she samples "all 31 flavors of Cuban dick" as her final "goodbye to Cuban sex" (42). Unlike in Cuba, however, where Adela must take political but not physical precautions with her sexual and gender expression, sex in the United States requires precautions against disease transmission. Adela is horrified when her sponsor, a gay Cuban nurse named Rolando, implores her to use condoms after seeing "something very scary" (47) at the clinic where he works. In a dramatic, full-page panel featuring an erect penis covered by a condom, Adela states:

> It's a total miracle that I obeyed and used condoms, because let me tell you straight up, I LOVE COCK. Just to say the word "cock" makes my mouth feel full. "Cock" is the only word as beautiful as "sista."
>
> Putting latex between me and good cock was a crazy ass idea to me, negative to me, not sexy to me. I had come to California and I wanted my sexual freedom and Rolando was telling me to use condoms???
>
> That queen was the only person in all the world who could convince me to use a condom. I listened and it saved my life. No drama. Just the truth. (48)

This panel is critical to the text's AIDS intervention work for several reasons. First, and most obviously, it is an erotic image of a condom, visually resignifying the latex barrier that Adela describes as "not sexy." Countering what Juana María Rodríguez calls the "imposed sexual abnegation evidenced in much mainstream AIDS prevention" (2003, 67), the panel acknowledges that prevention must affirm sexual desire.[21] But the text in the panel also refutes a teleological narrative that would depict Adela as moving from sexual repression to liberation, describing how the introduction of condoms feels like a denial of freedoms enjoyed in Cuba. By disrupting a facile journey-to-freedom narrative, the text invites readers to consider condom use as one risk-mitigation strategy among many and to contemplate the ways in which sex is always inherently risky, whether undertaken in a hostile political climate or in the midst of a pandemic. In this way AIDS is transformed from a singular, terrifying event that links sex to death into one of many sexual occasions requiring safety measures. Rather than predicating its safer sex message on disease fearmongering, in other words, *Sexile* presents sex as a pleasurable, mutually cooperative endeavor that is always imbricated in larger sociopolitical *and* biomedical risks.

It is important to acknowledge one sentence from this panel that might seem to undercut my argument: the words "I listened and it saved my life" present Adela as HIV-negative, thus potentially replicating the health-life/illness-death binary that I just critiqued. However, unlike health intervention texts that present and forbid a rigid litany of unsafe behaviors, *Sexile* presents Adela's involvement in behaviors associated with HIV risk, including sex work and drug use, and discusses how she minimizes that risk. She discontinues sex work, although its "pretty good benefits" include flexible hours and good pay, because "I was a great fuck but a lousy ho," but rather than stop using drugs she opts to "always respect the damage they can do and limit my use" (62). Adela's truncated sex work career, moderation in drug use, and embrace of condoms are presented as choices that work for her, but not as the only viable options for avoiding infection; the text thus invites contemplation of other possible risk-mitigation strategies.

Beyond its frank discussion of sex work and drug use, *Sexile* most insistently undermines the subject position of neutral expert that dominates health intervention literature through its treatment of the Mariel boatlift. Underscoring Juana María Rodríguez's point that HIV/AIDS service providers cannot assume "that all people want to live, that all of us are equally capable of negotiating sexual contracts, and that all of us benefit equally from health maintenance" (2003, 54), Adela's story engages its subject matter from the perspective of one who does *not* always want to live, does not negotiate sexual contracts from a position of equal power with her partners, and does not benefit from health maintenance. Adela's decision to leave Cuba is a painful one: "I had only one night. I packed my world into one bag, and rushed through my goodbyes. I touched every person I loved for the last time" (22). The text returns repeatedly to themes of separation and exile and to the trauma of being forcibly separated from a beloved family. Near the end, Adela discloses that the very same person who kept her alive by telling her to use condoms, Rolando, drank himself to death from the pain of exile. She herself confesses, in another dramatic full-page panel that depicts her naked (and still masculine) body swimming:

> Exile is a bitch, baby.
> You can't completely leave home.
> You're always still arriving home.
> Sometimes at night, you dream
> of your tired, lonely body
> swimming swimming swimming
> and wondering
> where the shore went. (50)

The emotional weight of this panel is established by the earlier images and discussion of the Mariel boatlift, through which Adela's own connection to Cuba is foreclosed. She can still talk to her mother on the telephone, but the Mariel images make clear the geopolitical and affective circumstances that keep her in a state of exile.

Although Adela's negative HIV status is implied in passing, it is not a primary element of *Sexile*'s plot. Rather than telling a story about how Adela avoids HIV infection, *Sexile* tells a story about how Adela reconciles herself to exile, separation from loved ones, and life in a gender-nonconforming body. As she puts it: "Some days I felt like the pain was going to swallow me up. I had this pain of being an exile, a transgender, and a sex worker. If I didn't take drugs, I would have been lost or maybe dead. Not pretty, but that was the real deal" (62). The happy ending to the text is not that Adela triumphantly declares her normative health status or stops using drugs but that she finds ways to live in and love her body despite her pain. The text underscores this when Adele revisits her dream of swimming. Here Cortez offers another full-page panel with a similar image of Adela swimming, this time in a much more feminine body, with long hair, breasts, manicured fingernails, and a penis. Adele states:

> I was swimming, swimming, swimming
> I had the fear like before
> Can't find the shore
> And then I knew
> All the in-between places are my home.
> This beautiful freak body is home.
> And every day I love it . . . (64)

This panel establishes that healing for Adela entails not maintaining a normative health status, not "passing" as a ciswoman, not reclaiming her connection to Cuba or declaring allegiance to the United States, but embracing the "in-between" status of her body (one that refuses the legibility of normative citizenship, gender, and health categories).

To conclude this section, I return to Hebert's preface to *Sexile*, in which he advocates for HIV/AIDS interventions focused on "the fullness of what we feel and the vastness of who we are becoming" instead of "tiny pieces of what we do" (2004, v). As a young adult in the 1990s, learning how to have sex in a pandemic, I remember often hearing (and probably at some point repeating) that HIV/AIDS is not about who you are but what you do. Although this message arose as a response to the homophobic characterization of HIV/AIDS as a "gay disease" and was believed to represent a tolerant, liberal approach to the virus, it actually served to amplify HIV/AIDS stigma by constructing the virus as a punishment for those who have sex in the "wrong" ways or use the "wrong" drugs. The fifteen years since *Sexile* was published have seen significant changes in HIV treatment: pre-exposure prophylaxis, in the form of drugs like tenofovir/emtricitabine (brand name Truvada), received FDA approval in 2012; antiretroviral therapy is now used not just to treat AIDS but to prevent HIV from developing into AIDS; and (at the time of this writing) the ACA means that many people previously without health care are able to access these medications. Despite these developments, however, the urgency of narratives asserting the value of lives like Adela's— lives that are nonconforming not only in terms of gender expression but also in terms of health behaviors—continues. The ongoing work of *Sexile* is not only to prevent HIV infection but to intervene in a range of circumstances that leave both HIV-positive and HIV-negative people unprotected against both infection and medical and social stigma.

Rafael Campo: Post-ACA Perspectives

The poetry of Rafael Campo offers a perspective overrepresented in medical sources on HIV/AIDS but underrepresented in literary ones: that of the physician. The son of a Cuban immigrant, Campo was a pre-med student at Amherst College in the mid-1980s when his English professor, Eve Kosofsky Sedgwick, encouraged him to keep writing poetry while pursuing a medical degree. After graduating from Harvard Medical School, he completed a residency in internal medicine at the University of California San Francisco

Hospital, working with HIV/AIDS patients. He remains both a physician and a poet. In his medical practice, he often treats immigrant, LGBTQ, and HIV-positive patients; in his poetic practice, major themes include health and illness. Spanning six original poetry collections and two essay collections, as well as a recent volume of selected and new poems, Campo's body of work represents not only the history of HIV/AIDS but also the history of efforts to create a national health care plan, from Bill Clinton's 1994 health care failure to the passage of the ACA.

Although Campo's writings critique the medical profession and normative understandings of health, they are—unlike the texts discussed previously—undeniably written from the position of someone whose life largely aligns with social norms. His poems and essays addressing HIV/AIDS show him grappling insistently with his identity as an HIV-negative, cisgender, monogamous gay man in a position of medical authority. This has led to a somewhat uneven reception of his work. In Latinx studies, critics appreciate his attention to middle-class identities, addressing what Elda María Román describes as the need to "challenge the assumption that the mainstream white experience is the normative middle-class experience" (2013, 13). Lázaro Lima observes that Campo's poetry "marks a discernible turn away from Latino poetry's emblematic emphasis on social protest toward poetry as the subversion of a privileged and reified language" (2007, 157); Ricardo L. Ortiz finds that "Campo exploits his medical training to refine into admirable precision the language in which he casts both his observations about his own medical work and his pointed critiques of the professional culture in which he performs it" (2007, 258). Within the health humanities, however, critics have expressed concern about the ethics of empathy in his work. Joanne Rendell worries that "his reverence of hybridity is in certain respects too transcendent, abstract, and equalizing" (2003, 224). For Lisa Diedrich, Campo's work risks appropriation, at times suggesting that "his patients' stories are his own, that they are, in fact, about him" (2005, 254).[22] However, most criticism on Campo, including the analyses just mentioned, tends to focus on the collection *What the Body Told* (1996) and his memoir *The Desire to Heal* (1998). In this analysis I examine two of Campo's HIV/AIDS poems of the post-HAART/post-ACA era, "Recent Past Events" and "Alternative Medicine," both published in his 2013 collection *Alternative Medicine*.[23] These poems reflect Campo's ongoing commitment to HIV/AIDS representation in a time when the pandemic has largely faded from public discourse.

Campo's work registers how the social and biomedical experience of HIV/AIDS has changed since the development of HAART, but it also reveals distressing continuities in the US health care system following the passage of the ACA. Campo's essay "Imagining Unmanaging Health Care"—an account of his time working as a resident in an HMO, published just four years after the failure of Clinton's efforts to reform the US health care system—reads familiar even now. "The more I have witnessed firsthand the inequities and the biases inherent in the current systems in place for the delivery of health care," he writes, "the less I have patience for the pre-approval forms for tests and utilization review decertification notices that appear in my patients' hospital charts—forms and notices through which M.B.A.'s tell me . . . how to practice medicine" (1998, 203). Campo's impatience in this passage makes visible a problem of the US health care debates that continues today: those who advance their opposition to universal health care conjure up the specter of a government-run health care system that will take away patients' "choices" even as the very system they defend places insurance administrators with business degrees—not doctors with medical degrees, and certainly not patients—in charge of health care.

Although *Alternative Medicine* gives less space to HIV/AIDS than Campo's earlier collections, "Recent Past Events" and "Alternative Medicine" occupy a particularly important position within it. The book consists of three sections, titled "Havana," "Alternative Medicine," and "Plonk." The first deals with themes of exile, belonging, and identity; the second with health and illness; and the third with personal relationships. "Recent Past Events" and "Alternative Medicine" are poems number eight and nine, respectively, of the nineteen poems that make up the middle section. "Alternative Medicine" is therefore not just the title poem of the collection *and* the title poem of its section, it is literally located (along with "Recent Past Events") in the physical center of the book. By centering HIV/AIDS in a collection that examines belonging, health, and love, Campo suggests that even as the virus continues to devastate lives, it also provides an occasion to reexamine our relationships with and responsibilities to one another and to craft health care policies that protect the most precarious. The advances in HIV/AIDS treatment combined with the stagnancy of national conversations about health care make Campo's later HIV/AIDS poems a particularly important site of analysis for my explorations of radical health.

The speaker of "Recent Past Events" returns to a theme visible in Campo's earlier writings on HIV/AIDS: survivor's guilt. For instance, in a personal essay from *The Desire to Heal* about his acquaintance with the Black gay writer Gary Fisher, who died of AIDS-related causes in 1994 in San Francisco while Campo was a medical resident there, Campo confesses his detachment from queer culture and activism: "Together and absolutely committed to each other from the beginning of our sexual lives . . . , my partner and I had become an inviolable (and hopelessly square) gay 'community' unto ourselves. Though I was elated to be in a place where gay people were more visible, I hardly knew personally any other gay men at all" (1998, 128). He writes, too, of a sense of guilt that prevents his friendship with Fisher from developing: "Not only did I woefully regret the hostility and the destructive impulses I had felt toward my patients with AIDS—the anger I harbored toward the epidemic itself having somehow been distorted and rechanneled through my sleep-deprived psyche toward those suffering in its wake—I also felt guilty for having been spared. . . . Some of my guilt was even less rational. I felt guilty for my monogamy, thinking myself too self-loathing to have become liberated sexually" (140–41).

The sense of survivor's guilt that pervades Campo's essay about Fisher also pervades "Recent Past Events," in which his speaker remembers the early years of the crisis:

> Some said we had their blood on our prim hands.
> We were ashamed of our good appetites.
> We marched together in gay pride parades.
> We feared their blood. We prayed for it to end. (2013a, 44)

Yet the ending of "Recent Past Events" takes a markedly different tone from the essays in *The Desire to Heal*. In the earlier text, Campo repeatedly recounts homophobic harassment he experienced throughout his medical training, from the colleague who whispers within earshot, "Can you believe it?—I heard he was gay. Too bad" (1998, 141) to the resident who smiles "almost smugly" (250) while aggressively questioning Campo's HIV status before scheduling him for a biopsy. By contrast, the final lines of "Recent Past Events" show that the speaker has seen gay rights enter the mainstream:

> We talked about adopting kids. We feared
> what people thought of us. We bought a house.
> We painted the back bedroom red like blood.
> We gave less money to the charities.
> We found a nice church that accepted us.
> The stained glass windows seemed miraculous.
> We ate our dinner. We remembered how
> we feared their blood, and how we prayed for it
> to end. And how it never really did. (2013a, 45)

Although these lines demonstrate that the speaker and his partner have achieved a kind of social legitimacy (homeownership, church attendance), HIV/AIDS stigma lingers in their fear of what others think. Furthermore, with its final line—acknowledging that the crisis has *not* really ended—the poem refuses a mainstream gay rights teleology that presents marriage, home-buying, and children as the culmination of queer activism. Its insistent use of "we" versus "them" language exposes how such a binary relies on understanding HIV/AIDS as a problem of others rather than as a collective sociopolitical concern.

Through its denunciation of homonormative complacency, "Recent Past Events" complicates the critiques by Rendell and Diedrich that Campo's poetry is marked by a "fantasy of empathy" (Diedrich 2005, 252) that too easily erases distinctions between Campo and his patients. The speaker repeatedly confesses feelings of shame and fear that distance the "we" of the poem from the "they." The strange enjambment of the final two lines also contributes to this distance: "we feared their blood, and how we prayed for it" aligns the speaker with religious rhetoric treating HIV/AIDS as an affliction of sinners who are the object of prayers from the morally upright, even as it also aligns him with desire for the communities most affected by the virus. "Recent Past Events," then, is an indictment of the purchase of gay respectability at the price of those marginalized by gay rights discourse, who remain unprotected. That the speaker's biographical details (long-term partner, upper-middle-class position, HIV-negative status) align with the poet's further sharpens its self-critique.

The poem immediately following, "Alternative Medicine," replicates the "we"/"they" distinctions that are such a preoccupation in "Recent Past Events." Subtitled "Wednesday Afternoon HIV Clinic," the poem consists of ten décimas, each with its own title, that offer snapshots of different patients at the clinic; the speaker of the poem is a health care worker.[24] Among the patients are an immigrant mother, a woman in an abusive marriage to an unfaithful man, and a medical skeptic. The relationships between provider and patient reveal varying degrees of intimacy and distance: the third décima, titled "Leukopenia," features a man who refuses to acknowledge his physician when out walking with his children; the seventh, "IVDU," features an intravenous drug user whose physician confesses, "I try/to hate him" (48); and the eighth, "Universal Precautions," features a museum worker who makes a point of asserting her commonality with her doctor, noting that she also wears gloves at work and provoking the thought that her "light touch might heal,/but in another sense" (48). In this way, the poem presents both a complicated portrait of HIV/AIDS, revealing the range of people living with its effects, and an interrogation of how the doctor–patient relationship is inflected with ideologies of race, class, gender, and sexuality.

These ten patient portraits are particularly useful for contemplating public rhetoric around HIV/AIDS and universal health care, as they work to disrupt narratives about innocence and guilt and to preempt questions about who does and does not deserve to access care. For many of the patients, no explanation is given for how they may have been infected. One, the patient in the fifth vignette ("Cardiomyopathy"), has managed to keep his viral loads undetectable even as his HIV-associated cardiovascular disease continues to progress. For others, behaviors are indicated that frustrate their doctors: the intravenous drug user; the woman who skips doses of her medication because she is afraid to reveal her serostatus to her husband; the person who rejects both antiretrovirals and processed foods and wishes that "all medicines came from the earth/and not some toxic lab" (49). By recounting the range of symptoms that the patients experience and the variation in their approaches to illness, the poem challenges the reduction of HIV/AIDS to simplistic stories and limited causal explanations, as well as its dismissal as a concern of gay men, sex workers, immigrants, and addicts. Faced with a disease that manifests in so many different lives, in so many different ways, what is needed is not interventions in health behavior but an intervention in the health care system, the crafting of health policy predicated on interdependence and an ethic of shared vulnerability, and agreement that everyone deserves medical care when ill, regardless of behavior, prognosis, or etiology.

Remedio

On March 9, 2020, just as COVID-19 lockdowns in the United States began, the *New York Times* ran a profile of Adam Castillejo, who had just revealed his identity. Previously known as "the London patient," the Venezuelan-born Castillejo had been declared cured of HIV the year before. Like "the Berlin patient" nearly twelve years prior, Castillejo had received a bone marrow transplant during the course of cancer treatment and was subsequently determined to be cured of HIV infection.[25] Having "realized that his story carried a powerful message of optimism," Castillejo declared: "I want to be an ambassador of hope" (Mandavilli 2020). Due to the spread of COVID-19, the story about Castillejo turned out to be the last feel-good medical news story many of us would read for a very long time. And the story is indeed full of good feelings, imbuing Castillejo with both health and heroism. He persevered through his initial HIV diagnosis in 2003, adopting "an unfailingly healthy lifestyle" (Mandavilli 2020); not even the discovery of a Stage 4 lymphoma diminished his "determination to spend whatever was left of his life fighting" (Mandavilli 2020). The article ends with an arresting image that captures Castillejo's heroism: "Having lost his lustrous dark hair several times over, he has now grown it to shoulder length" (Mandavilli 2020).

Without in any way downplaying the importance of the hope that Castillejo's case represents, I am skeptical of the hero narrative that the *New York Times* profile puts forth. Castillejo, described as "six feet tall and sturdy, with long, dark hair and an easy smile" (Mandavilli 2020), serves as a foil in the dominant HIV/AIDS narrative to Gaëtan Dugas, the Canadian flight attendant named as "Patient Zero" in Randy Shilts's controversial 1987 chronicle *And the Band Played On.* Due to Shilts's portrayal, Dugas is remembered as not only sexually promiscuous but also malicious, deliberately spreading the virus to hundreds of men. However, as Priscilla Wald points out, this portrayal turns Dugas—a historical person who ultimately died of an illness that was then poorly understood—into a vilified "narrative device" (2008, 232).[26] Healthy carriers of disease, according to Wald, are important characters in stories about contagious disease: "If the transformation of Gaetan Dugas into 'Patient Zero,' like that of Mary Mallon into 'Typhoid Mary,' demonizes the 'carrier,' it also humanizes the virus; it gives it agency and makes it comprehensible, attributing to it human emotions and responses" (234). Yet, as Wald has famously demonstrated, the impulse to turn the story of a disease into a narrative—replete with both villains and victims—has consequences that are not just biomedical but social and political.

Turning Castillejo into a personification of hope misrepresents important facts about how the HIV/AIDS pandemic is managed on a global level (not to mention how HIV infection is managed on an individual level). As the original *Times* report on Castillejo's case (published the year before and written by the same reporter) makes clear, bone marrow transplants are "unlikely to be a realistic treatment option in the near future" (Mandavilli 2019) due to their risks and harsh side effects. What will save the majority of people *now* living with HIV infection (as well as those infected in the near future) is not a spectacular *medical* event like a bone marrow transplant, but a spectacular *social* event: a revolution in the global health care system (making antiretroviral therapy accessible to everyone who needs it) and in the global economic system (ensuring that people have safe places to live, food security, and adequate resources to sustain a treatment regimen).

City of God, Sexile, and *Alternative Medicine* are not feel-good stories that proffer the hope of a miracle cure. And yet, I argue, *these* are the HIV/ AIDS stories we need now. Reading these texts in the fourth decade of a pandemic demands that we continue speaking of HIV/AIDS, as well as heteropatriarchy, white supremacy, and disease stigma, in the present tense. It requires that we recognize the work left unfinished from social justice struggles that we have declared over and complete, and that we remember those who gave their lives fighting them. Remembering these earlier Latinx histories of HIV/AIDS is particularly important because of how HIV/AIDS looms over contemporary debates around health care access. There is, first, the fact that universal health coverage is necessary for ensuring the protection of HIV-positive people now, whose access to life-preserving treatments depends on health coverage without economic barriers or exclusions for preexisting conditions. Second, the stories told by Cuadros and Campo of HIV/AIDS stigma and the story told by Cortez and Vázquez about resisting that stigma offer crucial insights for thinking about how health shaming surfaces in contemporary conversations about health care access. Recalling Gould's point that the HIV/AIDS crisis was allowed to flourish because those most affected were treated as "expendable" brings to mind how current conversations about the so-called obesity epidemic or diseases like diabetes inform debates about justice in the health care system. In the next chapter, I will explore in depth how diabetes makes visible the consequences of our collective failure to learn vital lessons from the HIV/AIDS crisis.

2

Sugar, Shame, Love

Diabetic Latinidades

Throughout the summer of 2020, as COVID-19 cases surged across the United States, the toll was particularly brutal in an area of the Texas-Mexico border known as the Rio Grande Valley (or colloquially as "the Valley"), where the death rate exceeded the state average by more than 50 percent (Solomon 2020). As the crisis intensified, the Valley received national attention. Sympathetic journalists (some with family ties to the region) sought to capture the cultural particularities of border life, an effort that unfortunately resulted in a collective emphasis on the role of the *pachanga* (an untranslated Spanish word, used in numerous articles, that means "party") in disease transmission. Edgar Sandoval (2020) of the *New York Times* wrote that "one thing that has continued to stymie efforts at keeping people at a distance in the Valley is its longstanding culture of pachangas, a colloquial expression for the festive family gatherings where social distancing is almost nonexistent," while Molly Hennessy-Fiske (2020; original emphasis) of the *Los Angeles Times* quoted Dr. Carlos Cardenas, chief executive of DHR Health, a hospital in Edinburg, Texas: "Anytime there is an excuse for our *gente* to have a party, a *pachanga*, we worry. . . . This virus is terrible for people with a culture like ours." Other factors contributing to the high death rate were relegated to the background: nearly one-third of the Valley's residents lack health insurance; the poverty rate in the region approaches 40 percent; few people in the area have the option to work from home; and Texas's Republican governor forbade local counties from enforcing stay-at-home orders.

Those familiar with the Valley had been warning about its COVID-19 risk for months. Sophie Novack, a health reporter for the independent, left-leaning *Texas Observer*, sounded the alarm in April 2020. Just a year before, Novack (2019) had written a powerful feature on the region's soaring rates of diabetic amputations, and she recognized that its diabetes caseload (triple the national rate) heightened vulnerability to COVID-19 across the region. Months before cases in the Valley began to climb, Novack spoke to the people she met while researching her earlier feature and filed a report that describes the safety dilemmas of those who rely on dialysis treatments (which require spending hours indoors with other patients each week), emphasizing the link between diabetes and complications from severe COVID-19. In hindsight, the quote she features from a volunteer at a local diabetes screening program is especially chilling: "We're going to have an incredibly horrendous situation here. . . . Tsunami, tidal wave, all those images. And we're not prepared" (Novack 2020).

Although the focus of this chapter is diabetes, I begin with this discussion of media attention to the COVID-19 crisis in a Latinx community because the relationship between the two diseases goes beyond the biomedical categories of comorbidity and risk. The two diseases are also linked representationally, as Latinx vulnerability in both cases is often explained in ways that emphasize cultural and biological traits over sociopolitical conditions. In the case of the Valley's COVID-19 crisis, the story across multiple media outlets of a "warm, close-knit family culture" (Sandoval 2020) in a place marked by "a slew of multigenerational households" (Solomon 2020), where "church, *pachanga* parties, and beach vacations" (Hennessy-Fiske 2020) predominate, illustrates my point. Although some apparently positive attributes surface in this narrative (like caring, supportive families), it is fundamentally a story that treats culture as a disease vector. In the case of diabetes, the stories are less compassionate, emphasizing genetic vulnerability, unhealthy Mexican food, and a culturally ingrained distrust of medical professionals. In fact, Novack's 2019 report on the amputation crisis in the Valley—as benevolently intended as it is—engages all of these tropes. In describing a conversation with one interviewee who had just learned that his blood sugar had spiked, Novack emphasizes that "Zamora's favorite foods are ones he has eaten his whole life: menudo, enchiladas, tamales," as though it were unusual for people to prefer the foods they grew up eating. She quotes a community health worker who states that it is "a typical thing with us, the Mexican people," to "believe other people and not their doctor" and imagine "that doctors only want their money" (Novack 2019), as though medical skepticism were not a common response to a capitalist health care system. Therefore, even though Novack does note economic inequality and lack of health insurance, and even though she demonstrates a personal sense of compassion for the people she interviews, her article ultimately suggests that the problem lies in innate Latinx racial difference: the Valley, as she explains, is "overwhelmingly Hispanic, a population that has a higher risk of developing type 2 diabetes" (Novack 2019).

Diabetes thus serves as an arresting illustration of the historian Natalia Molina's characterization of health as a "site of racialization" (2006, 15). Because diabetes is so closely correlated to lifestyle, those experiencing it are often subjected to public shaming that is both insidious and overt, treated by family members, acquaintances, employee benefits administrators, journalists, and even health professionals as responsible for their condition. Furthermore, this logic surfaces in rhetoric from both the right and the left. In response, Latinx cultural workers seek to imagine radical health in the face of a diabetes epidemic. This chapter begins with some thoughts about how diabetes might inform our evaluation of cultural theories of embodiment and risk (focusing in particular on Lauren Berlant's *slow death* and Rob Nixon's *slow violence*). From this meditation, I move into an analysis of texts (by Sonia Sotomayor, Tato Laviera, Virginia Grise and Irma Mayorga, and ire'ne lara silva) that simultaneously critique the social conditions that give rise to diabetes caseloads in Latinx communities and reject the stigma associated with a diabetes diagnosis.[1]

Slow Violence, Slow Death, and the Representational Challenges of Diabetes

Mainstream disability activists and scholars are fond of reminding those with enabled bodyminds that their corporeal/cognitive status is ephemeral, using the much-rehearsed refrain that *we will all become disabled if we live long enough*. Some disability activists refer to the nondisabled as TABS, a nickname derived from the acronym for *temporarily able-bodied*. Yet, as Jasbir K. Puar argues, the idea of disability as a universally shared future assumes race and class privilege: "Depending on where we live, what resources we have, what traumas we have endured, what color our skin is, what access we have to clean water, air, and decent food, what type of health care we have, what kind of work we do . . . we will not all be disabled. Some of us will simply not live long enough" (2017, xiv). She departs from more celebratory variants of disability scholarship that, as Alison Kafer notes, "often counsel an avoidance of stories that trace etiologies, mourning, or loss" (2016, 6). Instead, Puar interrogates "how disability is *produced*, how certain bodies and populations come into biopolitical being through having greater risk to become disabled than others" (2017, xix; original emphasis). The urgency of Puar's reframing came into sharp relief during the 2017 hurricane season, when two devastating storms—Harvey in South Texas and Maria in Puerto Rico—hit regions of the United States with large Latinx populations, leaving millions without power for protracted periods of time and endangering the lives of those requiring dialysis and those dependent on refrigeration for insulin injections.[2]

Such tragedies are only a particularly spectacular example of the everyday indignities that accompany experiences of diabetes. Diabetes is a devastating marker of the risk attached to specific bodies and populations, what Rob Nixon (2011) terms *slow violence* and Lauren Berlant (2007) calls *slow death*. Nixon's theory addresses "a violence that occurs gradually and out of sight, a violence of delayed destruction that is dispersed across time and space, an attritional violence that is typically not viewed as violence at all" (2011, 2), whereas Berlant's examines "the physical wearing out of a population and the deterioration of people in that population that is very nearly a defining condition of their experience and historical existence" (2007, 754).[3] Both slow violence and slow death are characterized by their imperceptibility, by their drawn-out evolution, by their lack of a single identifiable cause, and by the fact that they disproportionately affect marginalized communities. Although the two ideas are similar—and although the context for Berlant's work (the so-called obesity epidemic) might seem to make slow death an ideal analytic for this chapter—I ultimately find conceptual limitations in Berlant's theorization of slow death that affect its usefulness for this project and that merit extended discussion. For this reason, the analysis that follows relies more heavily on Nixon's slow violence, as well as on conceptual frameworks like slow living (Cvetkovich 2012) and slow care (Moran-Thomas 2019) that build on the work of both Nixon and Berlant.

The most obvious problem with slow death is what Lucas Crawford calls the "slender-normative" (2017, 448) language that Berlant deploys in its development. Others have criticized this language extensively (Love 2012; Luna 2016; Ward 2013), but I review its problems here. First, Berlant describes fatness, in and of itself, and absent other correlating health conditions, as a problem; they find "nothing heroic, promising, or critical" about fatness (2007, 767). Additionally, they describe fat as the result of eating "without an orientation" toward the future (779–80), thereby relying on the assumption that fat results from overconsumption of food (or consumption of the "wrong" kind of food) and ignoring substantial evidence that fat largely evades causal explanations (see Guthman 2011). As Heather Love points out, the major contribution of Berlant's theory is its "critique of the notion of sovereignty, which relies on an account of individual agency that no longer describes the situation of subjects under modern conditions of administration and management" (2012, 329)—a contribution that should preclude interpretations of it as mere victim-blaming. Berlant's work on slow death led to the book *Cruel Optimism*, which examines what happens when "something you desire is actually an obstacle to your flourishing" (2011, 1). Yet despite this critique, Berlant ultimately relies on erroneous understandings of fat as resulting from the behaviors of fat people, even as they question the link between individual behavior and individual agency.

I share many of Berlant's questions about agency. I am particularly interested in how the figure of the autonomous subject can rationalize racial health inequalities, resulting in what Anthony Ryan Hatch calls discourses of "biomedical individualism" that present "health as an individual moral responsibility" (2016, 104).[4] Berlant ostensibly seeks to resist appeals to personal moral responsibility, but the attribution of health disparities to behavior nonetheless makes the concept of slow death available for political uses that place both solution and blame on individuals. The idea that people's health reflects their behavior is not, of course, Berlant's alone; it also surfaces in liberal activism targeting food production and distribution systems. As the historian Charlotte Biltekoff reminds us, "despite seemingly scientific origins, dietary ideals are cultural, subjective, and political," such that "the process of teaching people to 'eat right' inevitably involves shaping certain kinds of subjects, and citizens, and shoring up the identity and social boundaries of the ever-threatened American middle class" (2013, 4).

Noting the uneasy coexistence of Berlant's critique of individual agency with a behavioral explanation of fatness, Love describes Berlant's work as marked by "blockages, dense conceptual knots that feel both personal and political" (2012, 332). My own method of unraveling these knots in this chapter is not to dismiss agency but to affirm the ways in which behaviors and choices that can seem unhealthy, counterproductive, or even harmful can, in fact, result from rational decision-making. In doing so, I attempt to work between analysis of the structural and analysis of the individual. While Berlant's critique of the sovereign subject and individual choice is one I find politically useful in some contexts, I am uncomfortable with its use to describe the behaviors of people who have long been presumed unable to make rational choices. For this reason, I propose that although it is important to be skeptical of rational choice, it is also important to keep in mind the political effects of that skepticism when considering the actions of people already assumed to lack autonomy. I recognize that my approach could simply seem to reverse the terms of Berlant's argument without resolving its tensions. I take this path because I suspect that the tensions are not resolvable. One way forward might simply be to assume the rationality of people often presumed to lack it, and to see what kinds of political possibilities flow from that assumption.[5]

The idea that "bad" choices are to blame for increases in both human body size and diet-related health problems undergirds health policy on both the right and the left. As Anna Ward (2013) points out, "obesogenic" explanations treating fat and its correlated health conditions solely as the result of environmental factors (like nonwalkable neighborhoods or a preponderance of fast food chains) "open the door for interventionist, paternalistic policies targeted at curbing consumption." As just one example, politicians on the left increasingly support legislation to limit serving sizes and increase sales taxes on the purchase of sugar-sweetened soft drinks. The most tangible effect of such initiatives is not to divert corporate profits to public health but to stigmatize individual beverage purchases and raise grocery bills. Meanwhile, on the right, biomedical individualism figures heavily in Republican opposition to the Affordable Care Act (ACA). Take, for instance, the remarks of Congressman Roger Marshall (R-KS) to the health website STAT in March 2017:

> Just like Jesus said, "The poor will always be with us." There is a group of people that just don't want health care and aren't going to take care of themselves. . . . I think just morally, spiritually, socially, [some people] just don't want health care. The Medicaid population, which is [on] a free credit card, as a group, do probably the least preventive medicine and taking care of themselves and eating healthy and exercising. (Facher 2017)

In this climate of health surveillance, the vulnerability of low-income people and communities of color to diabetes becomes construed as the reason why they should not be permitted to choose which foods to eat (or even to receive health care). It is therefore urgent to challenge the idea that behaviors resulting in poor health outcomes are *best* understood as a failure of rational choice and not as an occasion to examine the constraints under which *all* people make health-related decisions.

Another approach to the diabetes crisis—one I will not take here—might be to emphasize that diabetes, while *linked* to diet and lifestyle factors, is not *caused* by them; genetic and environmental factors also play a role. Yet there are also reasons to be cautious about such biomedical explanations. As medical anthropologist Michael J. Montoya notes, these explanations are often limited to genetics, despite the fact that "diet, physical activity, stress, labor relations, forced migrations, poverty, and a host of other sociohistorical factors shape and are shaped by experiences that can have biological outcomes" (2011, 31). For this reason, Montoya suggests that biological explanations can actually reinforce racialized diabetes stigma, "except in this instance, their behavioral inadequacies trigger their genetic ones" (85). These words of caution reinforce a core claim of *Radical Health*: that because *both* biomedical and cultural explanations of racial health disparities often reify racial hierarchies, we need aesthetic representations (and robust frameworks for interpreting them) to address the sociopolitical dimensions of health. In other words, I see art itself as a kind of health intervention because it expands our knowledge about the social conditions under which people make health-related choices and our ability to imagine a social order in which different choices become available.

This point about representation returns me to Nixon's concept of slow violence, even though the form of slow violence I discuss is distinct from the environmental degradation that prompted him to invent the term.[6] What strikes me about Nixon's book is that despite its title (*Slow Violence*), it is not primarily about the enactment of violence; rather, it is about *resistance to* violence, specifically about the actions of writers motivated by rage over "injustices they wish to see redressed, injustices they believe they can help expose, silences they can help dismantle through testimonial protest" (2011, 6). The writers and artists discussed in this chapter all, similarly, seek to address injustices caused not only by the devastation of diabetes in Latinx communities but also by the common (depoliticized) explanations for that devastation. Their work is characterized by impulses toward what Ann Cvetkovich (in conversation with Berlant) has called "slow living," or developing strategies "to live better in bad times" (2012, 168), and what Amy Moran-Thomas has called "slow care," or "ongoing and implicating joint work in the face of chronic debilitation" (2019, 25). In keeping with my argument throughout this book that Latinx expressive culture is in and of itself a health intervention, I pay close attention to the formal strategies deployed by the artists I discuss here, including the use of memoir, persona, theatrical monologue, epistolary essay, and the deliberate disarrangement of formal poetic structure. Ultimately, I argue that these texts offer a vision of radical health for those affected by diabetes, including those living under its diagnosis and those who care for them.

Diabetic Justice: Sonia Sotomayor

In an era when the composition of the United States Supreme Court has become a national obsession, the Puerto Rican Supreme Court justice Sonia Sotomayor enjoys a kind of liberal celebrity status, earning the affectionate moniker *Wise Latina*.[7] Yet although Sotomayor has long emphasized Latina identity as a crucial element of her public persona, in her career as a memoirist and children's book writer, she foregrounds another identity: that of diabetic. Describing her motivation to pen a memoir in the preface to *My Beloved World*, Sotomayor recalls a conference at which "a six-year-old asked plaintively if living with the disease ever gets easier" (2013, vii). In her first children's book, *Turning Pages: My Life Story* (2018), she lists her diagnosis at age seven as a formative experience from her childhood, along with learning English, hearing her Abuelita recite poetry, and mourning her father's death. Finally, she begins her most recent children's book, *Just Ask! Be Different, Be Brave, Be You* (2019), with a letter to readers that describes her childhood with diabetes: "Sometimes I felt different. . . . As I grew older, I realized there are many ways to be, that I was not alone in feeling different. I wanted to write this book to explain how differences make us stronger in a good way."

Before proceeding, I wish to note that I have no desire to contribute to what Lázaro Lima has called "the overwhelming and uncritical adulation" (2019, 3) of Sotomayor. Like Lima, I am skeptical of how her life story has been used to reinforce "the American dream of social mobility and the promise of democratic inclusion" (46). In particular, Sotomayor's account of her career as a prosecutor in both *My Beloved World* and *Turning Pages* betrays a troubling investment in US carceral regimes.[8] Even as I am mindful of these limitations, I believe that Sotomayor as a public figure prompts reflection on the differences between the political interventions of a Supreme Court justice and those of a writer. I argue that although her books often seem personal or even apolitical, their representations of diabetes offer an intervention in health politics at a moment of deep uncertainties about the health care system—an intervention that is substantively different from the one she will offer if the Supreme Court issues another ruling on the ACA.[9] Although Trump has vacated the White House, I write at a time when the ACA remains imperiled. In her role as a Supreme Court justice, Sotomayor possesses some capacity—certainly more capacity than most people—to influence whether and how the state might save or extend the lives of its vulnerable citizens. Yet in her role as a writer, Sotomayor makes a different kind of intervention, drawing attention to the everyday work of slow living in a sick and disabled body. For this reason, although I am skeptical of Sotomayor's possibility for staging a radical political intervention as a Supreme Court justice—given both her status as a minority vote on the court and the political path she followed in order to arrive on the court—I do see possibility in her cultural representations of diabetes.

That the themes of Latinidad and diabetes should intersect so prominently in Sotomayor's account of her life carries a significance that extends beyond her personal story. Here it bears mentioning that Sotomayor is a type 1 diabetic and that her condition is quite rare in Latinx communities (and in the US population overall) compared to type 2 diabetes. Because type 1 diabetes is an autoimmune disorder primarily attributed to genetics and type 2 diabetes is a metabolic disorder primarily attributed to behavior, type 1 diabetes is much less stigmatized than type 2 diabetes.[10] Yet Sotomayor refuses a political distinction between the types, declining to dwell on the etiology that differentiates her from the majority of the people who share her symptoms. Furthermore, she has been subjected to the racializing stigma and economic disadvantage typically associated with type 2 diabetes. For instance, Lima reports that on her confirmation Sotomayor was the most indebted sitting justice in the history of the Supreme Court, with "over $30,000 in debt, including medical bills not covered by her insurance plan"; this debt, he notes, was cast in racial terms as "'evidence' of her 'ethnic excesses'" (2019, 123). In 2017, Trump, whose signature accomplishments as president included the escalation of racist violence against Latinx populations and a drastic increase in the number of US citizens lacking health insurance, trolled his opponents with the prediction that he would ultimately replace Sotomayor on the court: "Her health. No good. Diabetes" (quoted in Swan 2017). Trump's comments are emblematic of a cultural logic that treats diabetics in general—and Latinx diabetics in particular—as unworthy of concern. As a writer, Sotomayor works against this logic in three crucial ways: by foregrounding the vulnerability of the diabetic body, by aligning diabetes thematically with other stigmatized illnesses, and by elaborating the ways in which diabetes has positively affected her life.[11]

Sotomayor emphasizes diabetic vulnerability through detailed descriptions of the work required to manage her diabetes. In *Turning Pages*, she describes the fear she felt on learning that she would need daily injections: "All those needles were scary!" (2018). In *Just Ask!*, she describes her insulin injections and then asks her young reader: "Do you ever need to take medicine to be healthy?" (2019). Finally, in *My Beloved World*, she offers a description of the daily effort required to maintain her health: "I test my blood sugar and give myself shots five or six times a day now. When deciding what I'm going to eat, I calculate the carbohydrate, fat, and protein contents. I ask myself a litany of questions: How much insulin do I need? When is it going to kick in? When was my last shot?" (2013, 278). More poignantly, she writes her diabetes into major life events, showing how it affects every aspect of her existence, even her wedding:

> I felt like a mannequin passed from hand to hand, until at the very end, when, with the cars already downstairs, their engines idling, I finally got a word in edgewise. We had forgotten one very important thing: I needed to eat something and have a shot of insulin. My mother froze in panic: whatever she had in the kitchen had disappeared in the comings and goings. So my cousin Tony ran to the diner across the street to get a turkey sandwich. I gave myself the shot and devoured the sandwich with a towel for a bib as the roomful of women screamed at me not to get mustard on the dress. (2013, 167–68)[12]

Together, these passages humanize a young girl facing chronic illness, ask nondiabetic readers to ponder their own need for medicinal interventions, and demonstrate the importance of attending constantly to chronic illness.

None of these passages directly mentions current debates over US health care policy, but all of them are deeply resonant at a time when millions of people face uncertain access to health care. For instance, although the phrase *preexisting condition* never appears in Sotomayor's books, both *Turning Pages* and *My Beloved World* instruct readers in the lived experience of having one, from the respective viewpoints of a young girl afraid of needles and a bride more focused on eating than on protecting her wedding dress from mustard. These passages do not shy away from the difficulty of chronic illness, but they are also humorous: Lulu Delacre's illustration in

Turning Pages of Sotomayor's feet sticking out from under a car (where she hid to avoid injections) is delightful, as is the mental image of Sotomayor eating a sandwich with a towel over her wedding dress. Finally, given the release of *Just Ask!* at a moment when insulin is at the center of national debates about the cost of prescription drugs, the question that concludes its section on diabetes ("Do you ever need to take medicine to be healthy?") functions as an ethical appeal to nondiabetic readers.[13]

Sotomayor's second strategy—the alignment of diabetes with other illnesses and disabilities—features most prominently in *Just Ask!* and *My Beloved World*. In *Just Ask!*, the character of Sonia is one of a group of multicultural children (Rafael, Anthony, Madison, Arturo, Vijay, Bianca, Jordan, Tiana, Anh, Julia, Manuel, Nolan, and Grace) who are planting a garden together; each describes a disability with which they live (asthma, mobility impairment, blindness, Deafness, dyslexia, autism, stuttering, Tourette's syndrome, ADHD, nut allergy, and Down syndrome). Sonia explains the title on the book's second page: "Kids are all different too. . . . Each of us grows in our own way, so if you are curious about other kids, just ask!" (2019). In interviews that accompanied the release of *Just Ask!*, Sotomayor describes being mistaken for an intravenous drug user in a restaurant bathroom, prompting her to confront a fellow patron and say: "Madam, I am not a drug addict. I am diabetic, and that injection you saw me give to myself is insulin. . . . If you don't know why someone's doing something, just ask them" (Balaban 2019). Yet although the title imperative of *Just Ask!* is implicitly directed at children who do not share the conditions described in each vignette (an interpretation reinforced by Sotomayor's description of the event that inspired the book), each child ends their segment by posing a question to the reader, who is presumed to not share their disability. For instance, Sonia asks the reader about medicines they have needed, while Anh—who stutters—asks: "Do you ever wonder if people understand you?" In this way, the book suggests that *all* bodies inspire questions, positing normative embodiment as a condition to be examined as much as disabled embodiment and promoting solidarity among corporeally variant and neurodiverse children.

In *My Beloved World*, Sotomayor offers an even more pointed intervention. Rather than disavowing a connection between stigmatized illnesses and diabetes (as when confronting the restaurant patron who assumes she is injecting herself with opioids), she explicitly aligns her diabetes with addiction: her father's alcoholism and her cousin Nelson's heroin dependence. The book begins with a prologue describing an argument between

Sotomayor's parents, with her mother insisting that she cannot be the only one to give their daughter insulin and her father insisting that his trembling hands prevent him from doing so. The outcome of the argument—that seven-year-old Sotomayor learns to give herself the shots—links the child's health management to that of her father: she presents his resistance to giving her the shots as arising from a concern for his daughter's safety caused by his own disease. Later in the book, she reflects on the addiction of her beloved cousin, whom she describes as "my inseparable co-conspirator" (2013, 16) and "my soul's twin, my smarter half" (252). In the years leading up to his death of AIDS-related causes, Nelson takes a steady job and starts a family but is unable to overcome his addiction, prompting Sotomayor to reflect: "I hadn't understood until then that one could be addicted to drugs and yet function normally in the world, holding a job and supporting a family. Nelson wasn't robbing people to get his fix; he wasn't shooting up in stairwells. He managed his addiction like a chronic disease, not unlike my diabetes" (251). Sotomayor's treatment of addiction as a public health concern rather than a criminal one aligns with a harm reduction model, although it is worth noting that she misses an opportunity to issue a more radical critique of criminality itself as a social construct (a missed opportunity that, overall, conforms with her early career in criminal prosecution).

The moving passages in which Sotomayor writes about her father's illness through the lens of her own diabetes also exemplify her effort to highlight positive effects of her illness. In one passage, Sotomayor reflects on how her life changes after her father's death: "I couldn't deny that our life was so much better now, but I did miss him. For all the misery he caused, I knew with certainty that he loved us. These aren't things you can measure or weigh. You can't say: This much love is worth this much misery. They're not opposites that cancel each other out; they're both true at the same time" (2013, 75). Strikingly, this passage about her father's love coexisting with the more debilitating effects of his disease immediately precedes a chapter in which Sotomayor elaborates the positive effects of living with diabetes. Here Sotomayor reflects on how her diabetes opened new career paths for her, first by putting her in contact with a woman doctor, "the first woman in a position of real-world authority I'd encountered" (76), and later by foreclosing the possibility that she might become a detective (since she is told that diabetics cannot become police officers) and causing her to dream instead of a career in law. (For a reader with a critique of carceral institutions that Sotomayor herself does not share, the exclusion from a law enforcement career is a particularly fortuitous development.) Especially moving are her musings, later in the book, on how her disease has made her friendships richer and more sustaining: "Learning to be open about my illness . . . taught me how admitting your vulnerabilities can bring people closer. Friends want to help, and it's important to know how to accept help graciously" (280). Both her flawed father and her diabetes, then, are things one cannot "measure or weigh"; both bring joy as well as difficulty, and both shape Sotomayor's remarkable life.

Just Ask! features an illustration by Rafael López that similarly conveys the coexistence of happiness and distress with which Sotomayor describes her life with diabetes. In this illustration, a child with light brown skin and short, dark hair, dressed androgynously in jeans and a T-shirt with pierced ears, sits in the center of a rose, inserting a hypodermic needle into their arm while a dragonfly buzzes nearby. As a powerful cultural symbol, the rose invokes beauty and love, and the child's facial expression—with closed eyes and a slight smile—appears relaxed and even blissful. However, the hand holding the needle is clutched into a tight fist, and the stalk from which the rose blooms contains thorns. The contradictions in this image strike me as particularly apt for capturing a complex portrayal of illness from a writer whose approach to disability and health I find both inspirational and limited. Like Sotomayor's words, López's illustration refuses to idealize or romanticize the disease but also insists on the value of those it affects—just as I myself have sought to insist on the importance of her representation of chronic illness without idealizing her.

In Remembrance of Tato Laviera

Characterized by its bilingual aesthetics and radical politics, the work of poet Jesús Abraham "Tato" Laviera Sánchez offers a contrast to that of Sotomayor.[14] Born in Santurce, Puerto Rico, in 1950, Laviera moved to New York's Lower East Side at age nine and lived most of his life in New York City. After establishing himself in the early 1980s as what Juan Flores called "a jewel of New York Puerto Rican expression" (quoted in D. González 2010) and publishing three critically acclaimed poetry collections, Laviera experienced periods of extreme health insecurity and economic precarity during the 1990s and early 2000s (culminating in an unhoused period in 2010) that resulted in long intervals without publishing. Of Laviera's health challenges, diabetes was the most damaging: he was diagnosed in 1984, experienced blindness and kidney failure as a result, and passed away at

Manhattan's Mount Sinai Hospital in 2013 at age sixty-three, after more than eight months in a coma (D. González 2013; Luis 2014). Partly because he claimed not to write autobiographical poetry and partly because he transitioned from writing poetry to writing plays after losing his eyesight, Laviera never to my knowledge addressed diabetes or blindness in his poetry (Laviera and Alvarez 2014, 288). However, he did attribute the shift in his writing to his blindness: "Tuve una transición de poesía a obra teatral porque yo era un taipiador de dos dedos. Cuando yo perdí la vista yo no podía taipear porque nunca aprendí . . . me adapté a trabajar con gente que me oye la voz y me taipean, de voz a dedo. Y esa transición hizo que se me hiciera más fácil desarrollar personajes o do other kinds of writing that I used to not like more than poesía porque la poesía es más personal" (Laviera and Alvarez 2014, 322).[15] Furthermore, his poetry from the very beginning has been interpreted as privileging oral rhythms over written words, and poems like "Word" (from his 2008 book *Mixturao*) that investigate the question of whether poetry is meant to be heard or read take on new valences when critics consider that they were written after losing his sight.[16] Finally, as Glenn Martínez (2014) has documented, Laviera was involved in diabetes activism and education near the end of his life. Here I examine the posthumously published "smile in remembrance of me," arguing that this poem offers insights into racialized experiences of diabetes even if it does not directly address the condition itself.

The poem "smile in remembrance of me" adopts the persona of a person who dies by drug overdose—a death, like those from diabetes, often attributed to personal failure—and offers a pedagogy for representing slow violence. Like Sotomayor, who depicts her diabetes as facilitating comprehension of her cousin's life with addiction, I suggest that awareness of the racializing effects of diabetes allows for a richer reading of Laviera's apparently unrelated poem. In "smile in remembrance of me," Laviera demonstrates how the death of his deceased speaker is treated as inconsequential. For Nixon, imaginative writing "can challenge perceptual habits that downplay the damage slow violence inflicts and bring into imaginative focus apprehensions that elude sensory corroboration" (2011, 15); Laviera gives a precise example of how this works. The poem's first two lines read as follows: "brothers, i died in silence—in screaming pain./now i nod eternally, smile in remembrance of me" (2014, 340). Whereas Nixon stresses the visibility/invisibility concerns at play in representing slow violence, Laviera characteristically turns to sound in order to juxtapose how the death appears from the outside ("in silence") against how it feels to the person experiencing it ("screaming pain"). Indeed, two symptoms of a heroin overdose mentioned here (inability to speak/"in silence" and appearing to doze off/"i nod eternally") produce the same representational problem that Nixon ascribes to slow violence; an opioid overdose is a violent event rarely recognized as such. As a result, the poem works to "complicate conventional assumptions about violence as a highly visible act" (Nixon 2011, 3) and to make apparent the violence contained within health crises that target specific populations (in the case of the poem, addiction; in the case of the poet, diabetes).

After addressing the physical symptoms that make a heroin overdose difficult to recognize, the speaker goes on to discuss the societal phenomena that make it difficult to mourn:

> overdose was not the cause of my death
> the cause of my death is this society we live in
> drugs is the international scheme of which i was
> only the receptive receptor,
> not the killer manipulator. (Laviera 2014, 340)

Here Laviera asks his readers to reexamine those deaths attributed to the negligence of the deceased (drug-related and, I would argue by extension, diet-related) in order to discern larger injustices. The reader is urged to "look around before you go to sleep, to/see if someone needs help on the empty staircase" (340), thus positioning the reader as witness to violence that does not seem violent.

Even as the speaker names "this society we live in" as the primary cause of his death, he does not depict himself as completely blameless: "brothers, besides my action that caused my death/as you look at my casket, look at the beauty in/me which i saw of you" (341). These lines emphasize that people who engage in self-harming behaviors still deserve to be remembered and mourned. Laviera's own comments about diabetes replicate this tension between accepting responsibility and addressing structural issues. In a 2008 interview with Martínez, Laviera attributes his own health decline to personal failure: "Nunca le hice caso a todas esas cosas . . . un descuido total" (quoted in G. Martínez 2014, 182).[17] Yet he also predicates his diabetes activism on countering a systemic failure of public health professionals to address Latinx communities in meaningful ways: "I started collecting all of these pamphlets and taking them to the community for people to read. . . . It was just information that was not culturally sensitive, not easy to read" (quoted in G. Martínez 2014, 183). In response, Laviera created the Diabetic Sugar Slam: a community-based performance art project offering people the opportunity to tell their diabetes stories in three-minute poems, songs, raps, or stories. Like the speaker of "smile in remembrance of me," who urges the reader to remember his "beauty," Laviera concluded that locating a definitive cause for the spread of diabetes in Latinx communities is less important than honoring the lives of those affected: "Everybody had a diabetes story. And those stories are actively in the community. . . . It was rampant and I decided to create music and art out of it" (quoted in G. Martínez 2014, 183).

When Laviera died, he was perhaps not as young as the speaker of his poem ("my death was a young death, and my body full of/life still" [2014, 340]), but it is nonetheless without question that sixty-three is also a young death. To read "smile in remembrance of me" and recall that it was written by someone who eventually died from a disease exacerbated by poverty and lack of consistent health care is an experience I find emotionally wrenching. As the speaker implores the reader to remember him smiling, I cannot help imagining the poet making the same plea to his own readers and admirers. Furthermore, as the speaker directs his brothers and sisters to "see if someone needs help on the empty staircase," I imagine the poet offering us, his living readers, similar instructions.

Performing Diabetes: Virginia Grise and Irma Mayorga

The Panza Monologues was written as a solo performance piece by Virginia Grise and Irma Mayorga while the two worked together at the Esperanza Peace and Justice Center in San Antonio, the script is now available in a scholarly edition with additional resources (like critical essays, author commentary, a glossary, and a DIY performance guide), and the authors also offer a limited-edition performance DVD. For the initial performances, Mayorga served as director and Grise as sole performer. With both artists now focused on other endeavors, theater companies currently producing the play have altered its format.[18] *The Panza Monologues* is both a revision and a critique of Eve Ensler's famous play *The Vagina Monologues*; like Ensler's work, it addresses gendered embodiment by examining a specific, stigmatized body part, but unlike Ensler, Grise and Mayorga seek to avoid gender essentialisms.[19] Both departures from Ensler's model are evident in the piece's title: first, its titular code-switch (substituting the English *belly* with the Spanish *panza*) indicates that the play will address racialized bodies; second, the piece's focus on the *panza* (a body part often imbued with gendered meaning but not directly linked to sex assignment) allows for a potentially trans-inclusive representation of feminine embodiment. Finally, unlike Ensler's piece, which aspires to represent a global experience of womanhood by incorporating monologues set around the world, Grise and Mayorga base their piece on interviews with Latinas in one geographic site: the central Texas city of San Antonio, a majority-Latinx city routinely included in listings of the "fattest cities in America."[20] As Grise and Mayorga describe the project in their introduction to the published script, the word *panza* "can be used with affection, a way to indicate that there's more of you around to love—especially around your midsection—or, cruelly, that you have a pot-bellied paunch for a stomach. . . . In our eyes, *panza* is a catalyst for looking at the social, political, geographic, and historical significance of women, of Latina/os, of ourselves" (2014, xxiii). This section will examine "My Sister's Panza," the monologue that most directly addresses diabetes.

"My Sister's Panza" is narrated from the perspective of a character who tells her "*panza* happy" sister's story (Grise and Mayorga 2014, 62). It opens by describing how the sister meets a man, falls in love, gets married, finds herself abandoned for a "thin little blonde" (62), and stops eating until "her *panza* began to shrink, pulled into her by the gravity of her collapsing heart" (63). Interspersed with this romantic history is another story about how the sister is diagnosed with diabetes at age seven. Although the critical response to *The Panza Monologues* has been mostly positive, the piece has also been critiqued; in a *Theatre Journal* review, Karen Jean Martinson writes: "The tough work of questioning the cultural practices that lead to obesity is somewhat underdeveloped in this piece that favors celebrating the overweight panza" (2005, 485). Monologues like "My Sister's Panza," however, confront weight-related health conditions in ways that are decidedly not celebratory. At the same time, the third-person narration from the perspective of someone (a sibling) who clearly loves both the main character and her *panza* enables Grise and Mayorga to balance this confrontation with a meditation on the harms caused by the stigma attached to fat and diabetic bodies.

The description of the family's encounter with the "doctor man" who gives the sister her diagnosis merits quoting at length:

> Our *mexicana* mother didn't know what he meant when he said we had too much of us around to love. . . . But, to save us, we had to change—everything. All our *comidas* had to change now, today, this minute! No more *tortillas de harina* smeared with butter, no more *Barbacoa* Sundays,

or *Arroz con Pollo* Fridays. No more *capirotada* piled five layers high. . . . But worst of all, they made *mamí* go to a nutritionist to learn how to cook out her love. They were teaching her how to lose the savings of our *panza* banks. Our *panzas*, they are what told her that her kids were 'never over her dead body' gonna starve. Even if we sometimes did. Mamí was crushed, broken. What had she done to her baby's pancreas? She didn't know, but she learned to poke my sister with life-giving shots to keep her *bebita* alive. (Grise and Mayorga 2014, 62)

This passage conveys an immense amount of information. First, the use of Spanish establishes the atmosphere of racialized distrust between the doctor and the family. In particular, the sentence "all our *comidas* had to change" contains an especially effective midsentence code-switch that conveys not only how the family understands its food practices as intimately linked to cultural expression but also how the doctor's criticism of the family diet is experienced as a cultural devaluation. More generally, the use of Spanish words for particular foods conveys the role of food in demonstrating intimacy and love in conditions of economic and social precarity, conditions that make changing diets a much more complex proposition than simply ordering a mother to change the way she feeds her children.

The mother's attachment to her children's *panzas* resonates with the work of social scientists, like Caitlin Daniels and Priya Fielding-Singh, who examine correlations between poverty and diet. Like the "doctor man" of the monologue, many middle-class people believe that poor parents simply lack the nutritional expertise to feed their children well; some, knowing about the lack of grocery stores in low-income neighborhoods and the lack of time that working parents have to prepare meals, are aware of structural causes for this correlation. But the connection between poverty and poor nutrition requires deeper analysis. For instance, because young children generally refuse new foods repeatedly before developing a taste for them, Daniels (2016) argues that use of familiar (often less nutritionally dense) foods constitutes a strategy to minimize food waste. Meanwhile, Fielding-Singh (2017) argues that food is a way to show affection that holds particular significance for parents who lack the means to give their children big-ticket items like name-brand clothing and vacations.[21] This research helps to explain why the mother is so "crushed, broken" by the health professionals' disparagement of her food practices: the doctor's instructions not only make it more difficult for the mother to feed her children but also pathologize one of her most accessible methods of expressing love.

Like Laviera's assertion that his health decline results from "un descuido total," Grise and Mayorga acknowledge the possibility of a dietary cause for the sister's diabetes; indeed, in their own comments on the script, they include "individual responsibility" among the factors that create a *panza*:

> Back in 2002–2003 we couldn't help but think that a predominance of obesity and poverty were somehow linked to the disenfranchisement of generations of Tejanas/os that has had an impact on our *cultura* economically, legally, spatially, physically, and also psychically. Our *panzas* were not only a matter of individual responsibility in regard to health and diet but also deeply connected to the material, spatial, historical, and embodied legacy we have lived as Tejanas. (2014, xxvi–xxvii)

This monologue makes clear that the mother's actions are not simply the result of ignorance. In making this claim, I am particularly mindful of a distinction between the way Daniels and Fielding-Singh characterize the dietary choices made by low-income parents (choices that minimize food waste and express affection under conditions of limited resources) and the way that Berlant characterizes them as mindless "comfort" in "insular households" marked by bleak circumstances in which "working life exhausts practical sovereignty" (2007, 779). I see the mother in "My Sister's Panza" not as exemplifying a counterproductive desire for comfort that limits her children's flourishing but rather as a person who makes the best choices she can in a situation of extreme constraint.

The monologue ends with lines that appear to mourn the sister's *panza*. The narrator informs us that her sister has stopped "eating until every roll of her *panza* was gone," all the while measuring her blood "to find sky-high readings of sugar, sugar, sugar" (Grise and Mayorga 2014, 64). As she looks at her sister, the narrator realizes that "you'd never know she'd even had a *panza* 'cause the sorrow of her hip bones pushed up against new, size 6 dresses she had to buy instead of 14's" and wonders bitterly "if the doctor would think she'd done enough to help control the sugar sweetness of her diabetes now?" (64). Instead of a story of weight loss as triumph, the narrator tells a story of weight loss as evidence of her sister's devaluation by lovers and health professionals alike. Noting that its principal character is no healthier at size 6 than she was at size 14 (with "sky-high readings of sugar, sugar, sugar" still present in her blood), "My Sister's Panza" alerts its audience to the problem of viewing weight as a proxy for health. The narrator does not evade the crisis of diabetes but insists that her sister's health challenges cannot be separated from a social context—represented by the doctor man and the unfaithful husband—that has treated her as unworthy of love and care.

Diabetic Love Song: ire'ne lara silva

Writing this chapter would not have been possible had Austin-based writer ire'ne lara silva not published the poetry collection *Blood Sugar Canto* in 2016. Dedicated to "everyone with diabetes and everyone who loves them," the book is an intimate and moving exploration of diabetes, covering everything from familial relationships to food injustice to sexuality to medical neglect, from the perspective of a diabetic Latina whose family and community are devastated by the condition. Throughout, as literary critic Amanda Ellis observes, silva "imagines illness experiences mired in and marked by an oppressive unevenness of power and pain" (2021, 177). The poet explains her vision in an interview with *Rogue Agent Journal*:

> The more I wrote the more clear it became that what I wanted to do was write a book that would . . . make people with diabetes or other chronic illnesses feel less alone. A book that might help non-diabetics glimpse what diabetes meant in a life. A book that would help family members or community members establish a dialogue. A book that might make doctors and other health professionals understand their patients a bit better or treat them more humanely. A book that would share my particular experience—a woman of color, Mexican-American, Indigenous, queer, from the border, born in poverty, an artist—living with diabetes. (silva 2017)

Blood Sugar Canto is composed of five sections, each containing at least one poem dedicated to an emotional experience like despair, shame, or love; one poem addressing access to nutrition and medical care; and one poem engaging the relational aspects of the disease by examining how diabetic speakers address their parents, lovers, siblings, and health care professionals. In this way, silva presents diabetes not simply as a medical condition but as a corporeal experience with emotional and political dimensions.

I conclude this chapter with an extended analysis of *Blood Sugar Canto* because the collection as a whole exemplifies my argument in *Radical Health* for Latinx expressive culture as a health intervention. In particular, the collection instantiates the acts of slow care that Moran-Thomas locates in communities ravaged by diabetes, the labor of "trying to stave off bodily loss and failing organs day in and day out, year in and year out, over and over again" (2019, 25). For Moran-Thomas, stories of diabetes are a crucial element of slow care: the "slowly told tales of individuals' daily struggles to live with lasting conditions" (95). She invokes the Latin American literary genre of the *crónica* (a nonfiction narrative that unfolds in installments) to describe these stories of slow care, noting that while English separates "two distinct terms and ideas—*chronicle* (a slow-building written account) and *chronic* (a slow-progressing condition)" (95)—the Spanish word *crónica* can evoke both a narrative and a disease. Although my fellow literary critics might quibble with my description of the poetry collection *Blood Sugar Canto* as a *crónica*, given that the term is most often associated with prose narrative, I find Moran-Thomas's reformulation of the term (via the discipline of anthropology) as a slowly unfolding story and disease that produces the labor of slow care particularly well suited to silva's collection. Rather than exploring a single poem, then, this final segment of the chapter will address *Blood Sugar Canto* as a whole by examining three larger themes: diabetic feelings, modes of care, and radical health.

Diabetic Feelings

Two years apart, in 1978 and 1980, two women writing in very different literary traditions, both in treatment for breast cancer, asserted their right to be unhappy. Susan Sontag's "Illness as Metaphor" notes that when people are "encouraged to believe that they get sick because they (unconsciously) want to, and that they can cure themselves by the mobilization of will," the effect is to blame the ill: "Patients who are instructed that they have, unwittingly, caused their disease are also being made to feel that they have deserved it" (2001, 57). Similarly, Audre Lorde's *The Cancer Journals* dismisses the notion that "no truly happy person ever gets cancer" as a "monstrous distortion" that "does nothing to encourage the mobilization of our psychic defenses against the very real forms of death which surround us" (1997, 76). Although narratives of cancer and diabetes differ in some aspects, the perception of a link between bad feelings and ill health persists.[22] Berlant argues that obesity and associated health conditions can be explained by the ways in which "the scene of slow death . . . makes vague the relation of life as health, life as something worked toward" (2007, 779). Here, illnesses linked to weight (like diabetes) result from an affective orientation toward health that presents itself as "resignation" to the "consequences" of insalubrious food consumption. This belief is not Berlant's alone; as Crawford points out, Berlant relies on a common assumption that "trauma makes one eat more, eating is what 'causes' fatness; fatness is therefore a manifestation of that trauma" (2017, 452). The problem here is not just the selective logic (as Crawford notes, trauma also causes people to eat less and lose weight) but also that it makes it more difficult to talk about the unhappiness of diseases like diabetes. Acknowledging this problem in the context of breast cancer, Lorde boldly invites the accusation that her anger has caused her disease: "Was I wrong to be working so hard against the oppressions afflicting women and Black people? Was I in error to be speaking out against our silent passivity and the cynicism of a mechanized and inhuman civilization that is destroying our earth and those who live upon it? . . . In this disastrous time . . . what depraved monster could possibly be always happy?" (1997, 76–77). In a similar vein, silva devotes considerable space to the bad feelings of living with racialized diabetes.

A quick perusal of the table of contents of *Blood Sugar Canto* offers a striking number of poems indexing negative emotions: "song for fear," "despair, you are invited to my table," "*susto*," "*soledad*," "depression: an interrupted sestina," and "shame: a ghazal in pieces." As noted, these poems are distributed throughout the collection; there is no emotional arc through which the collection begins in despair and ends in joy (or vice versa), suggesting that to live with chronic disease is to live with difficult feelings. Furthermore, the poems in which silva most self-consciously experiments with form all address negative emotions. For instance, "depression: an interrupted sestina" begins with six fairly traditional six-line stanzas before collapsing into four stanzas that disintegrate the form, each consisting of five to seven lines containing no more than three words each, only to conclude with the expected triplet; the form of the poem mimics the experience of living with episodic depression in which periods of relative emotional composition are interspersed with periods of intense decomposition. The opening and closing lines of the poem reflect this interpretation; the speaker opens by asserting that "no one said the darkness only subsides/never disappearing never dying" (silva 2016, 71) and ends by urging an interlocutor to "breathe slowly in-between wait till it subsides" (72). Meanwhile, in "shame: a ghazal in pieces," silva uses the repetition of the ghazal to convey the negativity directed at her fat brown body while also conveying a sense of indignation so intense that she cannot contain it within a recognizable poetic (or even grammatical) form: "who are they to name your body my body a shame body shame my weight shame your weight shame how i look shame how you look shame my disease shame my story say we have made ourselves sick we keep ourselves sick" (73). In an interview about this poem, silva (n.d.) describes her writing process as follows: "I let the ferocity I felt explode the ghazal structure while retaining the ghazal-inspired language."

In the first section of the collection, in a poem titled "despair, you are invited to my table," silva articulates the need to find a way to live with negative emotions. Here the speaker invites despair to share a meal, acknowledging that they already share a life: "you have my eyes you have my mouth/we have my face we have my hands/i speak with your voice you touch with my hands" (2016, 18). The importance of this acknowledgment is underscored in the title of the opening section, "speak with your voice touch with my hands," taken from this poem. The speaker goes on to tell her despair that she has given up "fighting you declaring that you didn't exist" and instead wishes to "find a way to live peacefully with our same face" (18). The poem thus introduces an orientation toward negative emotions—often assumed (as Sontag and Lorde illustrate) to cause illness or to interfere with healing—as ever-present companions whose presence is not always welcome but who cannot be rejected. Rather than seeking to overcome these feelings, silva's speakers seek to live with them without wholly succumbing to them.

This exploration of the despair that accompanies chronic illness can, at times, appear to sit uneasily not only with cultural mandates for the sick to maintain a "positive attitude" but also with the dominant feeling—pride—of mainstream disability activism. The poem "*susto*," for instance, explores both biomedical theories of a link between diabetes and stress as well as Mexican folk wisdom that attributes illness to *susto* (sudden fear). In this poem, silva writes: "the old women say it is the accumulated weight/ of so many *sustos* that cause diabetes/*susto*: not fright but trauma/and stress and shock and loss and grief" (2016, 51). As Puar might argue, poems like this one are firmly "anchored . . . in the lived experiences of debilitation" and therefore "may not represent the most appealing or desired versions of disability pride" (2017, xxiv). Nonetheless, as Ellis, who explores the role of *susto* in silva's earlier work, asserts: "These stories matter . . . now more than ever because the U.S. economy is increasingly globalizing privatized trade and, therefore, globalizing susto. Here, our understanding of illness and healing must shift to recognize the ways larger forces make us structurally vulnerable to illness and trauma" (2017, 55).

The greatest challenge in *Blood Sugar Canto* to a politics of disability pride occurs in the poem "en trozos/in pieces," which addresses fear of amputation. This poem recounts the amputations that have occurred in the speaker's family as a result of diabetes: her maternal grandmother's toe; her Tía Lupe's toes, feet, legs, and finally fingers; her father's feet. The speaker says that what her father "feared most was to go in pieces./now i fear it too" (silva 2016, 40). These lines about the fear of amputation may be irreconcilable with disability pride, but I argue that they advance a vision of disability justice that seeks not just to celebrate disability but also to understand its causes.[23] For this speaker—who inherits generations of medical neglect—justice resides not only in the creation of wheelchair ramps for family members who have experienced amputations but also in access to treatment for those who have not (yet). Furthermore, the poem shows that these two goals are not mutually exclusive; it ends with the speaker declaring her love for her body: "oh body *cuerpecito mio*/how many years i wasted not loving you/judging you for what they said you lacked/for what you were too much of/too big too dark too fat too short too *india* . . . oh body *cuerpecito mio*/i will never see you through their eyes again . . . i will learn to take care of you/as i have learned to love you/no terror no terror/only love" (41). What is important here is the speaker's refusal to qualify her love for her body. She does not say, *I will take care of you so that you will not undergo amputation.* She simply resolves to care for her body, suggesting a commitment to love her body in any shape it takes.

Modes of Care

Throughout this chapter, I have emphasized the structural forces that render particular populations vulnerable to diabetes. In so doing, I have sought to reframe common understandings of choice, arguing that while diabetes can be understood as causally linked to certain kinds of lifestyle choices, these choices need to be understood within their sociopolitical context. Rather than exclusively scrutinizing the health behaviors of low-income people of color, I argue, we should also scrutinize the circumstances in which those behaviors take place. At the same time, I cannot set aside the fact that there is an enormous discourse of blame around diabetes, a discourse to which people living with the condition are not immune. I have already noted, for instance, how even the diabetes activist Tato Laviera attributed his own declining health to personal "descuido." In my own experience teaching the work of silva in Latinx studies classes, I find that my students—the majority of whom are Latinx and from Texas—routinely invoke relatives and friends with diabetes who "don't take care of themselves." silva does not sidestep this discourse of blame and care but addresses it directly, through poems that engage both biomedical care (the experience of visiting doctors) and sociopolitical care (the social and political structures that offer or deny support for the care of diabetic bodies).

Of these poems, "'we don't give morphine for heartburn'" and "grace," in particular, address relationships with health care providers. The first describes an experience in which the speaker's brother, "a young brown-skinned man with scars and tattoos" (silva 2016, 29), goes to four different doctors in excruciating pain and is turned away each time, assumed to be drug-seeking, with the words "we don't give morphine for heartburn." On his fifth visit to the emergency room, a doctor finally admits him to the hospital, schedules him for surgery, and offers a diagnosis: "he was diabetic and had high blood pressure/and high cholesterol" (29). As with Laviera's "smile in remembrance of me" and Sotomayor's *My Beloved World*, which I read as a record of the ways in which addiction and diabetes, particularly when experienced by young men of color, are subject to similar stigma, the poem balances its representation of stigma with an assertion of the value of the brother's life: "i am grateful every day i didn't lose him/i am grateful that we went back and went back and insisted and insisted" (30). In the poem "grace," which follows seven pages later, the speaker goes to a medical appointment and is filled with shame when the physician's assistant asks her to remove her shoes, immediately apologizing "for not having had a pedicure" (37). She is shocked when the assistant treats her feet "gently and respectfully" (37), a new experience after "years of them wincing and trying/not to touch my skin with their gloved/hands, my still strong and sensitive feet made ugly" (37). Here adherence to basic professionalism is experienced by the speaker as a gift: "as humble/and great a gift as if she had washed my/feet with her hair" (38). While it might be tempting to read these two poems as examples of good doctor/bad doctor, the power of "grace" comes from the fact that the experience it describes is not typical of the speaker's experience in doctors' offices. (It is also significant that the professional in this poem is not a doctor but a physician's assistant.) The two poems together, then, depict the cumulative effects of gender, race, and class in medical settings and critique health professionals' disregard for racialized diabetic bodies. These poems demonstrate that just as the behavior of patients is influenced by larger structural forces, so too is that of medical professionals, such that efforts to reform the profession must focus beyond the individual.

The poems "*dieta indígena*" and "*tequilita,*" address diet and its connection to diabetes. The poem "*dieta indígena*" begins by asking "what would we be if we were still/what our ancestors ate" and ends with a plea to "let us eat what our ancestors ate/decolonize your diet *mi raza*/it is time to regain our strength" (silva 2016, 23).[24] Meanwhile, the comma in the title of "*tequilita,*" frames the poem as a letter to a lost lover; the speaker recalls joyous times when "we rampaged from one coast to another, in south texas, on the other side of the border, in austin and san antonio," but also notes that "after that doctor's visit, i left you and never looked back" (52). Of all of the poems in the collection, these come closest to offering dietary advice and, if read in isolation, could be seen as putting forth a behavioral explanation for diabetes. However, it is important to note that "*dieta indígena*" devotes four stanzas to a description of how colonialism and capitalism have altered the American food production and distribution system over the past five centuries ("500 years and our bodies . . . cannot thrive on a diet of chemicals/and preservatives/sulfur dioxide sodium benzoate sodium nitrate/propyl gallate BHA BHT" [22]); by contrast, only the final stanza describes "food which can renew our health/food we can grow with our own hands . . . *chile frijoles tomates aguacate calabaza/nopales chayote* cacao amaranth quinoa" (23). Meanwhile, in "*tequilita,*" the speaker personifies tequila and assigns to it active verbs ("it's been five years, four months, three days since you last touched my lips" [52]; "you made the lights, the singing, the dancing all the more beautiful" [52]); "*tequilita,*" concludes with the narrator offering thanks to the beloved: "i thank you, *tequilita,* for keeping your distance" (54). Both address the reasons why people might not be able to make the same choices, including the colonization of food production and addiction. Like Grise and Mayorga, who use Spanish words to communicate their characters' emotional ties to particular kinds of food, silva also uses code-switching in these poems to imbue certain foods with love; in "*dieta indígena,*" the objective is to convey an ancestral bond with unprocessed foods, whereas in "*tequilita,*" it is to convey affection for tequila, showing that changing one's diet (even when desired) can entail loss and mourning. Together, these poems critique the way the food industry makes people vulnerable to diabetes while also addressing the ineffectiveness of merely prescribing dietary changes.

Finally, "diabetic epidemic" addresses how diabetes has proliferated among particular populations and devastated entire communities within the span of a single generation. The poem begins with the line "*la azucar* we heard it whispered first" and ends with a plea: "why is *la azucar* still being whispered/we should be screaming it" (silva 2016, 31). Recalling Laviera's use of sound and Nixon's concern for the conditions under which violence becomes perceptible, the poem juxtaposes the whisper against the scream in order to pose the question of when its titular epidemic will receive the attention it deserves. In the first stanza, the speaker tells us, "at first it was only the old people" (31); in the second, she relays that "then it was my father" (31); in the third, "years passed and then it was everyone's grandparents" (31); in the fourth stanza, even as more and more people are diagnosed, the speaker conveys that "i went to college and learned nothing at all about it" (31). As the poem progresses, the stanzas themselves get longer and longer, first because the lines are longer and then because silva adds more lines to each stanza, thus making the increase in caseloads visible on the page itself. Meanwhile, the stanzas bring the disease closer and closer to the speaker, from "the old people" to her father to "everyone's grandparents" to "my brother my youngest brother" (32), and finally herself:

> i changed my diet gave up drinking
> thought i'd managed not to become a target
> no one told me not sleeping and skipping meals and stress
> and living on adrenaline could tear the body down
> or that insulin resistance was part of polycystic ovarian syndrome
> and then that day came the confirmation from the doctor
> (silva 2016, 32)

In this poem, silva presents "a violence that is neither spectacular nor instantaneous, but rather incremental and accretive" (Nixon 2011, 2) and grapples with what it will take to make others recognize and care about it. Moran-Thomas asserts that if "slow violence is difficult to discern, slow care might be even harder to see: meal by meal, gesture by gesture" (2019, 284). The meals and gestures chronicled in the poems I have discussed in this section bring slow care to life.

Radical Diabetic Health

To conclude, I turn to the book's title poem: "blood•sugar•canto," which exemplifies my argument by presenting the diabetic Latinx body as a site of structural injustice but also as socially and politically valuable. The first half of the poem rehearses many of the themes already discussed in its description of living with diabetes as a "constant battle of/necessity versus necessity" (silva 2016, 63). The speaker offers an excruciating list: "a box of syringes/vs/gas money/the price of sufficient insulin/against/the cost of groceries/testing strips and lancets/vs/the light bill/the cost of one healthy meal/vs/the cost of three fast food meals/another co-pay/and another co-pay/vs/the cost of not seeing the doctor" (63–64). Against those who would place the blame for diabetes on those living with the disease, silva's speaker insists that "it is not as simple/as/eat this not that eat that not this/take this not that take that not this/do this not that do that not this" (65). The poem thus reminds us to direct our critical scrutiny not at those living with diabetes but at the social conditions that force people to make untenable choices. Yet for this speaker, diabetes is not only about poverty and medical neglect but also about acquiring a new relationship to one's body. The poem insists on the importance of "learning to listen/to *your body* and to *your blood* . . . you learn to listen/until you are the one writing the song/ and the daily challenges are the discordant notes/you must work into the score/making something more beautiful/than what was there before/not planned not wanted/but more powerful/because it is truth" (65). These are, of course, the lines that give the poem its title, that evoke the blood sugar canto of the collection. Using the metaphor of song to describe diabetes, silva is not downplaying its devastation or celebrating its occurrence. Rather, she is reminding us that illness is an important and unavoidable part of life; it constitutes the "discordant notes" of the canto of our lives, the "daily challenges" that make the entire song more beautiful: "not planned, not wanted, but more powerful because it is truth."

Imagining diabetes as music requires loving the diabetic body, loving diabetic communities, believing that those most affected deserve the best possible resources to care for their bodies. To enact the love that allows this music, this blood sugar canto, to do its work requires working against powerful cultural scripts. Again, I quote from "blood•sugar•canto": "i know/no one said/we were worthy of love/no one said/we were precious/or that our lives were gifts/no one said/let us learn to love ourselves" (silva 2016, 66). The love evoked in these lines stands in powerful contrast to the biomedical individualism that undergirds our most common narratives about the proliferation of diabetes, an ideology leading to the conclusion that some people simply do not deserve to receive health care, an ideology that cannot be our only means of understanding diabetes in a social world structured to make all of us more vulnerable to it and some of us particularly so. Of note in these lines are the plural pronouns used by the speaker, pronouns that provide a contrast to the singular language of neoliberal individualism that dominates public discourse around health: *we* are worthy of love, the speaker tells us, *we* are precious, *our* lives are gifts. silva insists that the love that contests diabetes must be collective and communal. For silva, reimagining diabetes is not merely an aesthetic exercise but a process of unlearning the isolating language of neoliberal health care and biomedical individualism, the social narratives that portray entire communities as undeserving of health and undeserving of love. "blood•sugar•canto" is one effort to discover a new song to replace these destructive and damaging stories. I have no words better than those of silva, so I will end this segment with her lines: "i will begin here/with these lines/learning love/one utterance at a time . . . i will make song" (66).

Remedio

More than any of the other health disparities addressed in this book, diabetes seems to spur contemporary audiences to action. At public presentations on my research for this chapter, over and over, attendees asked me what *we* can do to stop this disease. I was unfailingly struck by the urgency of the question but always uneasy answering it. We need universal health care, I would say—*real* universal health care, covering our entire population and not excluding the undocumented or those whose choices some find objectionable. We need to stop disparaging people's food choices and radically reimagine food access. Making these recommendations, I was always painfully aware that I sounded like a literary critic: not enough legalese, not at all politically feasible. There was always someone in the room with more knowledge of political procedure and tax loopholes than I have.

What was particularly difficult about these interactions was the sense that some people would come to my talks expecting advice about how to stop consuming sugar, advice of the sort that appears in the best-selling diet exposés of Gary Taubes (2011, 2016) and David Leonhardt's *New York Times* (2016, 2018) opinion pieces. Taubes and Leonhardt offer critiques I sometimes find useful about corporate neglect for people's wellbeing, even as their advice is predicated on liberal ideas about individual sovereignty that I (like Lauren Berlant!) find undertheorized and naive. I think, for instance, about how tobacco profits have ultimately been unaffected by cigarette taxes or by the push to make smoking socially unacceptable; cigarette manufacturers simply began marketing their products in low-income communities and throughout the Global South (Maloney and Chaudhuri 2018). The health risks of smoking have been displaced to locations where people have fewer financial resources to deal with the negative health outcomes associated with smoking; these are the people keeping the tobacco industry in good health while the industry itself contributes nothing to *their* health. How will the effects of taxing soda be any different? How is it possible that the sugar industry is not already carefully recording these lessons? I have begun to imagine sugar as another product that will, eventually, become so stigmatized among middle-class consumers that candy-and-cereal eaters, like cigarette smokers, will be banned from partaking of their habits in public areas (like the university campus where I work) and forced to pay higher health insurance premiums (as they do on my employer's health plan).

When I'm not standing in front of large rooms of people trying to parse through these questions, I'm actually very glad to be a literary critic. When I pick up my copy of *Blood Sugar Canto* and piece together thoughts for the ending of this chapter, the one thing I know I want to say is that it is art's emphasis on the speculative that, to my mind, makes it the best resource available for considering these questions. As a literary critic, I'm so glad I have the luxury of focusing not on what I believe to be politically feasible (like the soda taxes that seem to gain more and more political support every day) but on what I believe to be right: that we have to find a way to make it possible for everyone to nourish their bodies as best as they can, and to provide health care for everyone when their bodies fail (even if we disagree with how they choose to nourish their bodies). We have to stop asking what it is people have done to make themselves sick, or what they have done to make themselves poor. I don't know what it will take to end diabetes, but I do know that diabetes will not end until we believe that people with diabetes—particularly the racialized poor—deserve to live. And I fervently believe that art has a role to play in valorizing the lives of those currently deemed undeserving. In the next chapter, I continue this thought experiment to consider the role of art in fostering new modes of support for survivors of domestic abuse.

3

Healing without a Cure

Radical Health and Racialized Gender Violence

Performance artist, disability justice activist, poet, and writer Leah Lakshmi Piepzna-Samarasinha insists on the radical potential of abuse survivors' stories but also critiques the literary conventions often used to make them legible. In the preface to their own memoir, *Dirty River: A Queer Femme of Color Dreaming Her Way Home*, they distinguish their narrative from the best-known abuse and survivor narratives: "This book is not *The Courage to Heal* and it's not *Push*. It's not *When You're Ready* or *No: A Woman's Word* or any of the other brutal, pastel-covered incest books of the lesbian, feminist '70s and '80s. It's not an incest horror story book, and it's not palatable, either. In the end, I don't get normal. I get something else" (2015, 15). In essays published after *Dirty River*, Piepzna-Samarasinha further reflects on the absence of disability in many survivor stories as well as on the "deep parallel between the way being a survivor is seen only as a fault, never as a skill, and the way ableism views disabled people as individual, tragic health defects" (2018, 232). This chapter takes up Piepzna-Samarasinha's insistence on both the power of survivor narratives and the need to read such narratives critically.

Inspired by Piepzna-Samarasinha's desire "to explore my survivor wounds and knowledges . . . *as a disability narrative*" (2018, 166–67; emphasis added), I argue that Latinx representations of gender-based violence contribute to the theorization of radical health developed throughout this book. Just as Piepzna-Samarasinha dreams of survivor stories that offer "less pain" without "bleed[ing] into the ableist model of cure" (2018, 231), *Radical Health* is about a search for wellbeing not predicated on the possession of normative health status. This chapter examines texts that prompt us to imagine radical health after abuse in ways that don't pathologize victims (or perpetrators) and that present heteropatriarchal violence not as an "individual, tragic" event but as embedded within larger systems.

Even after decades of feminist organizing, individualized framings of gender-based violence are inscribed in the terms most often used to name it: *domestic abuse* and *intimate partner violence* both imply aggressions contained within a home or limited to the participants in a romantic relationship. This narrow view has disastrous consequences for how such abuse is understood. Despite general public sentiment that abuse survivors deserve empathy, victim-blaming persists through widespread perceptions of domestic violence as rooted in individual behavior (aggressors' choices to engage in abusive acts and survivors' willingness to tolerate them) instead of as an instantiation of health injustice unfolding in a context of gender and racial terror. Survivors *in the abstract* are not (overtly) blamed; however, those who do not involve law enforcement are seen as not serious about stopping the violence, those unable to protect children from abusive partners are treated as unfit parents, those fighting back are viewed as "just as abusive," those remaining with or returning to abusive partners are said to exercise poor judgment, and those forced to rely on an abuser for economic or physical support are seen as pathologically dependent. The privileged victim is thus one who trusts law enforcement, has no children affected by the violence, never engages in self-defense, and possesses the economic and physical means to leave. In short, to be a sympathetic survivor requires being able-bodied, middle-class, gender-conforming, a citizen or authorized immigrant, and racially coded as white.

My thinking about the role of expressive culture in reframing gendered abuse is informed not only by Piepzna-Samarasinha's disability justice theory but also by the work of Black feminist sociologist Beth E. Richie and Chicana feminist cultural critic Rosa-Linda Fregoso. Richie, for instance, claims that literary texts by writers such as Toni Morrison, Alice Walker, and Maya Angelou advance a more comprehensive account of violence against Black women than the work of many mainstream social scientists regarded as experts on the topic:

> [These texts] are suggestive of a more contextualized, nuanced under-standing of the experience of male violence in the lives of women, an understanding that is consistent with a Black feminist theoretical ori-entation. They describe an experience of abuse that is embedded in a cultural rhetoric, a set of racialized experiences and particularities of community and social conditions that links intimate partner violence much more closely to public policy and community violence than does the dominant white feminist analysis found in the contemporary social science literature. (2012, 148)

In a similar vein, Fregoso asserts the importance of cultural representations in responding to violence, arguing that although "the global proliferation of gender-motivated violences may be rampant and overwhelming, it is not a closed narrative, but a contested one" (2006, 110). In the following pages, I examine journalistic, musical, and literary texts by Sonia Nazario, Alynda Mariposa Segarra/Hurray for the Riff Raff, Manuel Muñoz, Rigoberto González, and Angie Cruz, attending to how each creates (or forecloses) new narratives of gender violence.

These texts are part of a much larger body of Latinx expressive culture, including canonical texts (like Sandra Cisneros's 1992 short story "Woman Hollering Creek" and Esmeralda Santiago's 1997 novel *América's Dream*) and experimental ones (like Carmen Maria Machado's 2019 memoir *In the Dream House*), that addresses intimate partner violence. I chose the texts discussed in this chapter for two reasons. The first has to do with how each artist presents the sociopolitical context that foments heteropatriarchal violence, including US military interventions in Latin America, restrictive immigration laws, state divestment from low-income racialized commu-nities, and cultural logics that devalue feminized bodies of color. Second, I selected texts whose endings challenge "the idea of cure as the only way to heal from abuse" (Piepzna-Samarasinha 2018, 232). The disability scholar Eunjung Kim reminds us that "cure, even at the individual level, does not always provide relief" (2017, 9) and notes the particular violence of cures that emphasize individual over societal transformation. Of course, the cure most often promoted in domestic violence narratives is the unequivocal separation between survivor and abuser, an outcome that can be messy and difficult (if not downright impossible) for many to achieve. None of the texts

I examine in this chapter ends with such a separation, even though books with such endings have played a key role in my own survival, because of my choice to focus on texts that complicate the idea of cure.[1] Together, the texts discussed in this chapter prompt a response to violence that aligns with the notion of radical health that I advance throughout this book: a collective enterprise linked to larger sociopolitical structures, one for which individualized rhetorics of personal accountability are insufficient.

Radical Health and Heteropatriarchal Violence

The turn in this chapter to gender violence as health injustice marks a shift in my line of argumentation. Whereas the previous chapters examined stigmatized health conditions, this chapter and the one that follows use health and disability as analytics to examine social concerns that are both pervasive in contemporary Latinx expressive culture and infrequently addressed through health or disability frameworks. Making this leap requires stressing the distinction between *medicine* (the treatment of individual bodies and health conditions) and *public health* (the promotion of community wellbeing). To understand intimate partner violence through the lens of radical health requires a comprehensive reassessment not only of individual behaviors but also of larger social formations: immigration control, law enforcement, the social safety net, and cultural narratives that affirm (or devalue) women and gender-nonconforming people of color. It also requires emphasizing that to frame domestic abuse in terms of health is *not* to suggest that either survivors or perpetrators are individually sick.[2] Rather than pathologizing individuals, I seek to excavate the cultural narratives that surround gender violence in order to move beyond what Piepzna-Samarasinha calls the "harsh binary of successful and fixed or broken and fucked" (2018, 232). Key to this endeavor is not just the text itself but also the interpretive tools used to examine it. For this reason, before discussing my chosen texts, I offer comments about the terms and theories that are central to my work.

As noted, terms commonly used for relationship violence and those who experience it are all imperfect. *Domestic violence* and *intimate partner violence* are the most widely recognized terms, but when used exclusively, they reinforce the idea that the causes of such abuse are confined to the private sphere. Therefore, although I use both because of their legibility, I interchange them with other terms. For instance, I use *heteropatriarchal violence* to emphasize that such violence is not solely perpetrated by men against women but is rooted in heteropatriarchal social formations and broadly targets feminine, nonbinary, queer, trans, and otherwise gender-nonconforming people. My preferred term is also the clunkiest (and thus the one I use least): *racialized gender violence* not only captures the gendered nature of the violence I describe but also conveys how white supremacy affects the experience of such violence. In addition, *victim* and *survivor* both have benefits and drawbacks for designating those who experience abuse. The term *survivor* is often preferred by activists seeking to avoid the stigma attached to the label of victim. Yet, as literary critic Sarah Ropp points out, survival is a "highly individualistic" (2019, 132) concept correlated to the ableist discourse of overcoming. Writing of her own experience of sexual violence, the writer and cultural critic Roxane Gay asserts:

> I am marked, in so many ways, by what I went through. I survived it, but that isn't the whole of the story. Over the years, I have learned the importance of survival and claiming the label of "survivor," but I don't mind the label of "victim." . . . I don't want to diminish the gravity of what happened. I don't want to pretend I'm on some triumphant, uplifting journey. I don't want to pretend that everything is okay. (2017, 20–21)

Gay's account of her decision to use the word *victim* alongside *survivor* resonates with feminist scholarship advocating a more expansive vocabulary. As Theresa A. Kulbaga and Leland G. Spencer write: "We reject the victim/survivor binary as false, . . . and we believe that both terms can be valuable and meaningful in context" (2019, 12). For these reasons, I use both.

My engagement with the work of Richie and Fregoso also requires further discussion. Although their emphasis on the role of culture in retheorizing racialized gender violence makes them logical interlocutors, it is worth noting that my focus on multigender, US-based Latinx writers removes their work from its original context: Black women's experiences of violence (Richie) and feminicidal violence in Latin America (Fregoso). Richie does not directly cite the Combahee River Collective's famous declaration that if "Black women were free, it would mean that everyone else would have to be free since our freedom would necessitate the destruction of all the systems of oppression" ([1983] 2000, 270), although she does credit the collective as formative for her development of a Black feminist response to violence. Still, her premise—that unless our understandings of gender violence center the experiences of the most vulnerable, we will not be able to end it—aligns with the collective's insight that liberation must address the experience of the most oppressed. In this spirit, Richie offers her Black feminist anti-violence framework to address the circumstances of other marginalized survivors: "I would even go so far as to argue that a Black feminist analysis of male violence . . . would extend benefit to women whose circumstances seem to be quite different from the women whose stories frame the central argument of this book. Take, for example, the issue of male violence toward non-Black, Latina immigrant women" (2012, 161). In using Richie's work in this chapter, I take up her invitation to extend its reach.

Whereas Richie reminds us of the public nature of domestic abuse, which is shaped by community norms and public policy, Latin American and Latina feminist scholars like Fregoso who engage with feminicide, or feminicidio—the murders of poor Indigenous, Black, and racialized women throughout the Americas—note that public regimes of racial and gender terror are also lived intimately in the domestic sphere. This body of scholarship is best known as an effort to explain the deaths and disappearances of women in Ciudad Juárez, Mexico, which began to receive sustained attention in the late 1990s; scholars of femicide have expanded their analysis to address racialized gender violence throughout the Americas. Fregoso and coauthor Cynthia Bejarano note that "feminicide bridges the 'private' and 'public' distinction by incorporating into its definition *both* systematic or structural violence sanctioned (or commissioned) by state actors (public) and violence committed by individuals or groups (private)" (2010, 8). Mexican feminist Marcela Lagarde y de los Ríos offers a definition of *feminicidal violence* that accounts for "the violent deaths of girls and women such as those that result from accidents, suicides, neglect of health, and violence" (2010, xx). Richie, Fregoso and Bejarano, and Lagarde y de los Ríos all insist that gender-based violence is perpetuated in the home, in the community, and by state-based institutions; it targets victims through direct physical brutality as well as through emotional manipulation, resource deprivation, and systemic neglect.[3] For this reason, the most effective response to heteropatriarchal violence will not be a solely individual one, focused on punishing or incarcerating perpetrators and rescuing victims, but a communal one that takes into account histories of intergenerational violence, including violence within the home and state-sanctioned or community violence.

The texts I discuss in this chapter present different forms of violence that frequently intersect. Nazario describes how gang and narco violence link with domestic violence in Central America, addressing the state neglect and US immigration policies that allow both to flourish; Segarra emphasizes the intersections of racial and gender violence; Muñoz and González depict how intimate violence inflicted on queer men of color is enabled by misogynistic violence against women; Cruz and González consider how US military and economic interventions and border enforcement policies foment abuse. As I will make clear in my individual analyses, I am much more a fan of some of these texts than others. Considered together, however, they reveal the urgency of reconsidering the frameworks that we use to theorize racialized gender violence and offer strategies for contesting it.

Sonia Nazario: An Abuse Melodrama for the Trump Era

Raised in Argentina and the United States, Sonia Nazario is a Pulitzer Prize–winning journalist who has worked for the *Los Angeles Times* and is now a contributing opinion writer for the *New York Times*. She is widely known for her 2006 bestseller *Enrique's Journey: The Story of a Boy's Dangerous Odyssey to Reunite with His Mother*, which follows the route taken by a Honduran teenager seeking reunification with his mother in the United States. Based on a series of stories that Nazario wrote for the *Los Angeles Times* in the early 2000s, *Enrique's Journey* received a Pulitzer Prize; has been adopted as a common read by universities, cities, and high schools across the nation; and was adapted for young adult readers in 2013. Although it was published nearly two decades ago, the book garnered renewed attention after 2014, when media attention began focusing on unaccompanied Central American minors entering the United States. As Monica Hanna notes, the book has "afforded Nazario a platform from which to critique US migration policy to a US audience" (2016, 369), one that took on new importance after Donald Trump assumed the US presidency in January 2017 and began implementing punitive measures against Central American asylum seekers: separating migrant children from their parents, moving to preempt their asylum claims, and slashing aid to their home countries. Drawing on extensive experience reporting from Honduras, Nazario responded to these moves with a series of opinion pieces for the *New York Times* about the conditions that motivate Central Americans to seek asylum in the United States, focusing on violence against women, gang warfare, and the political corruption that foments both. Most of these are short editorials; two are long-form reports accompanied by photo essays from Victor J. Blue: "'Someone Is Always Trying to Kill You'" (Nazario 2019b), about gender violence, and "Pay or Die" (Nazario 2019a), about gangs and corruption.[4] I begin my discussion of Latinx representations of heteropatriarchal violence with a discussion of these essays, including my concerns about how they portray gender violence in Central America, for two reasons. First, they illustrate the urgency of examining the representational strategies used to depict violence; and, second, they are the most widely distributed of the texts under consideration here and reflect dominant ideas about gender violence in ways that that highlight the interventions of the other texts.

Although *Enrique's Journey* has been embraced for what Marta Caminero-Santangelo calls its efforts to encourage "readers to 'identify' with migrants" (2012, 160), it has also drawn criticism. Hanna and Caminero-Santangelo both note that the book casts blame on mothers who migrate and then send for their children. Ana Elena Puga characterizes *Enrique's Journey* as a "migrant melodrama" (2016, 73) that depicts "undeserved suffering by innocent victims as the implicit price of inclusion . . . in a new nation-state" and that treats suffering as the currency by which migrants purchase "rights that should be universal and have sometimes already been granted, at least on paper, by international or national laws" (75).[5] Nazario's recent *New York Times* articles mitigate some of the problems with *Enrique's Journey*, showing the untenable situation in Central America that motivates migration, but also heighten the emphasis on suffering as the basis for migrants' claim to asylum. As a result, these articles not only make a spectacle of Central American women's pain in ways that reinforce a larger narrative of Central American criminality but also undermine claims to protection made by other migrants and survivors of domestic abuse. When magnitude of misery becomes the basis of a claim to safety, then others who endure less implicitly become less deserving.

Nazario's articles feature explicit images from interviews with women throughout Honduras and at a detention center in Adelanto, California. The nature of these images means that a content warning is in order: in the rest of this paragraph, I will replicate and analyze Nazario's descriptions of violence against women; readers who might be traumatized by these descriptions should skip to the next paragraph. The editorial based on interviews at Adelanto exemplifies Nazario's approach. Her description of the experience of a Guatemalan woman, Mayra Lucrecia Arriola Hurtarte, contains specific and brutal images that underscore Puga's critique of her sensationalistic representation of migrant suffering:

> She said he regularly choked her until she passed out. He would cut himself and make her drink his blood. She showed me the fingers he had broken. She raised her blue uniform to reveal two letters—the first two of his name—that her husband had carved into her belly.

It got worse. She said he stuffed his hand up her vagina, saying he was trying to pull her womb out. Another time he held her down and rammed a knife up her vagina. (Nazario 2018a)

In "'Someone Is Always Trying to Kill You,'" based on interviews conducted in Honduras, Nazario includes similarly brutal descriptions to illustrate both the magnitude of the violence and the experiences of individual women. Early in the essay, she explains: "Honduras is one of the world's deadliest places to be a woman—a 2015 survey ranked it in the top five countries, with El Salvador and Syria. . . . And the ways they are being killed—shot in the vagina, cut to bits with their parts distributed among various public places, strangled in front of their children, skinned alive—have women running for the border" (2019b). Many of the individual stories are accompanied by images from Blue's accompanying photo essay. The story of how Heidy Hernández was terrorized by her husband is paired with a picture of Ms. Hernández in a wheelchair, prominently displaying legs that have been amputated just below the ankle and just below the knee, staring past the photographer, with a caption that reads: "Heidy Hernández lost her feet and part of her right leg after her husband attacked her with a machete" (2019b). That of Sonia Fuentes, shot twelve times by her ex, is accompanied by a photograph of a woman with the top of her shirt open to reveal bullet-shaped scars on her upper chest (2019b). In Nazario's articles, women's bodies as objects of violence are displayed graphically and repeatedly, through both text and photograph.

Nazario's purpose, it merits emphasizing, is to elicit empathy for migrant women. Yet these images call to mind María Josefina Saldaña-Portillo's warning against a focus on "the most extraordinary and horrific testimonies" that can "feed pornographic mythologies of the criminalized nature and barbaric sexuality of the Central American enemies we must keep out, consequently confirming the need for the very territorial and epistemic borders" (2019, 3) that exacerbate migrants' oppression. They further demonstrate what Saidiya Hartman has called "the difficulty and slipperiness of empathy" (1997, 18) as they risk "fixing and naturalizing this condition of pained embodiment" (20). I will return later in this chapter to Hartman's critique of empathy, but for now I wish to note simply that Nazario's detailed depictions of migrant women's suffering are deployed in order to condemn the inhumanity of asylum policy under Trump and to propose alternatives that she presents as more just, more humane, and more fiscally responsible. Indeed, following Puga's theorization of the migrant melodrama, it could be argued that Nazario is re-creating the very form of the asylum petition itself, placing her readers in the position of judges who decide the fates of these women: "Demands for performances of suffering are also written into the language of international and national laws that mandate, for instance, that one prove a 'well-founded fear of persecution' in order to be granted asylum" (Puga 2016, 75). Still, the onslaught of brutal images in Nazario's editorials effectively reduces Central American women to objects of violence.

Although she occasionally alludes to the history of political conflict in the region (a history that implicates the United States), Nazario emphasizes cultural explanations: "It's about machismo—the culture of which goes back to colonial times, when conquering Spaniards came without wives and treated the indigenous like slaves. Today, in a world ruled by gangs and narco groups, it's about engendering maximum terror in your enemies" (2019b). By offering a cultural explanation for violence against women in Central America that vaguely reaches to the deep colonial past without mentioning much more recent historical events that have shaped the current political climate in Honduras, Nazario minimizes the context for that violence and pathologizes the region. By contrast, sociologists Cecilia Menjívar and Olivia Salcido find that such explanations for gender violence can work against advocacy for survivors by reinforcing "the notion that gender-based abuse does not need the state's intervention because it is part of a group's culture" (2002, 901).

Unlike Nazario, scholars and legal experts studying feminicides in Central America emphasize the history of US military intervention in the region, including support for military governments in Guatemala and for the Intelligence Battalion 3–16 in Honduras, that deployed violence against women as a military strategy. In this framework, violence against women is the result not of a violent culture but of a political history that links the United States and Central America. According to attorneys Angélica Cházaro and Jennifer Casey, throughout Guatemala's civil war (1960–1996), a "generation of young men forcibly recruited to the army were indoctrinated in the use of sexual violence as a weapon" (2006, 151). For Guatemalan attorney and human rights advocate Hilda Morales Trujillo, contemporary feminicidal violence raises "specters of the forms of gender-based violence committed during the armed conflict" (2010, 127). Nazario is not unaware of this context. However, her scant mentions of US interventions in Central America actually seem to absolve the United States of culpability: "Thanks to the contra war, when the United States secretly funded right-wing militia groups in Central America, there are an estimated 1.8 million guns in Honduras. And yet one in 10 female murder victims are strangled to death" (2019b). It is unclear what Nazario's point is here, and the relationship between the two sentences is curious: Nazario's use of the phrase "and yet" implies that the staggering number of guns in Honduras, a direct result of US military aid, has nothing to do with the number of women being killed. But the statistics she cites imply the opposite: an unspecified number of women—possibly as high as nine in ten—are being killed with guns.

Nazario's case for granting these women asylum mobilizes three arguments: (1) that the relatively small number of Central American domestic abuse survivors seeking asylum can easily be accommodated by the United States; (2) that granting asylum to Central American women with a credible fear of gender-based persecution need not lead to open borders; and (3) that supervised release of asylum seekers while their claims are being processed is more cost-effective than locking them up in for-profit detention facilities.[6] All of these claims are, in fact, true. But they raise additional questions: What if the number of individuals from Central America currently seeking asylum in the United States *weren't* "reasonable"? (Certainly, some of Nazario's readers already believe this.) Why *not* argue for open borders—or at least, for rewriting US immigration law? What if indefinite detention—a known cause of psychological harm—were the cheaper option? Ultimately, Nazario's line of argumentation opens the door to assessing asylum claims based on the magnitude of suffering and to denying asylum claims not believed to be reasonable and cost-effective. The ethical reasons to grant these women asylum (including the role of the United States in creating the violent conditions in which they live) receive much less attention in her work.

More than ten years ago, writing about feminicide in Ciudad Juárez, Alicia Schmidt Camacho argued that the crimes resulted from "a wholesale inability to imagine a female life free of violence" (2005, 267); Nazario's articles, which purport to advocate for women experiencing violence but trade in the spectacle of that violence, betray the same inability. One defense of Nazario's approach might be that she is using the rhetoric that she believes to be most persuasive. Is a time of escalating xenophobia like our current moment, one might ask, *really* the right moment to make political claims for asylum seekers based on radical Black and Latinx feminist theory? Isn't Nazario right to make arguments the average *New York Times* reader will find compelling and sympathetic? The problem with this logic is that by framing gender violence primarily as interpersonal violence rooted in a uniquely misogynistic culture, Nazario contributes to misunderstandings of it. In fact, it is worth noting that Nazario's columns were written in direct response to the efforts of the Trump regime, in particular former attorney general Jeff Sessions, to classify domestic violence as "private" and thereby declare Central American women fleeing it as ineligible for political asylum (Benner and Dickerson 2018). Sessions's opinion conceded the "harrowing experiences" of women like those profiled in Nazario's articles but nonetheless insisted that they constituted "general hardship" (US Department of Justice 2018) rather than political persecution. Even though the United Nations High Commissioner for Refugees has advocated an asylum category specifically for domestic abuse survivors (United Nations High Commissioner for Refugees 2004) for two decades, the *political* nature of gender-based violence has not been definitively codified into US immigration law—nor is it clearly stated in the work of high-profile migrant advocates like Nazario.[7]

What Nazario's articles prompt me to ask, then, is what kind of representation might promote—in the slightly altered words of Schmidt Camacho—the *ability* to imagine a feminized life free of violence? What is needed in the place of Nazario's anguishing images is an accounting of racialized gender violence that makes clear how—as Piepzna-Samarasinha, Richie, Fregoso, and others have demonstrated—the physical, sexual, and emotional violence experienced by multiply marginalized women and gender minorities is rarely limited to the household but is enabled and escalated by community norms and public policy (including foreign policy, military interventions, and immigration policy). In search of such accountings, I turn to texts that facilitate a much more comprehensive understanding of heteropatriarchal violence.

Alynda Segarra/Hurray for the Riff Raff: Settling Delia's Score

Alynda Mariposa Segarra is the founder, front person, and songwriter of the band Hurray for the Riff Raff; they are the group's only member to perform on all of its recordings.[8] Before the 2017 release of the concept album *The Navigator*, discussed in the conclusion to this book, Hurray for the Riff Raff was best known to Americana music fans (a genre for which I confess a soft spot). Because *The Navigator* engages more directly with Segarra's Puerto Rican heritage than their prior work does, it has been hailed as a claiming of identity; music critic Jim Farber (2017), for instance, writes in the *New York Times* that Segarra's earlier recordings reflect an "internalized cultural exile" and that it was only with *The Navigator* that "Segarra finally took full ownership of her heritage." I dispute this interpretation, arguing in particular that the song "The Body Electric" from Segarra's 2014 album *Small Town Heroes* (an album that, by the way, features the Puerto Rican flag on its cover, contradicting the claim that Segarra did not "take full ownership" of their heritage until releasing *The Navigator* three years later) exemplifies a Latinx feminist approach to racialized gender violence. To support this contention, I focus on the song's apparently simple lyrics and on Segarra's performances at live shows, on social media, and on video.

"The Body Electric" is an answer to the folk genre of the murder ballad, which Segarra makes clear with the line "Delia's gone, but I'm settling the score." The line refers to "Delia's Gone," a particularly famous example of the murder ballad genre, versions of which have been recorded by Johnny Cash, Bob Dylan, Pete Seeger, Waylon Jennings, and Harry Belafonte, among others. According to an entry on the true crime website *Murder by Gaslight*, which bills itself as a "compendium of information, resources and discussion on notable nineteenth century American murders," the song is based on the 1900 domestic violence murder of Delia Green, a fourteen-year-old Black woman, in Savannah, Georgia (Wilhelm 2010). As music critic Ann Powers (2014b) writes, the idea for the song came to Segarra when they noted how often musicians and fans alike "would regularly sing along with choruses about killing women, comfortably accepting gender-based violence as part of the ballad tradition." In keeping with this tradition, the song's lyrics are sparse and repetitive. The verses describe threats and acts of violence by men ("Said you're gonna shoot me down, put my body in the river . . . He shot her down, he put her body in the river") and responses, which include both complacency ("the whole world sings like there's nothing going wrong") and action ("I said, 'my girl, we gotta stop it somehow'") (Hurray for the Riff Raff 2014b). Meanwhile, in each chorus, the singer asks a variation of the question: "Oh, and tell me, what's a man with a rifle in his hand/gonna do for a world that's so sick and sad? . . . Oh, and tell me, what's a man with a rifle in his hand/gonna do for a world that's just dying slow?" While the description of violence is repetitive ("shoot her down, put her body in the river"), it is not particularly graphic; the lyrics offer no details about the victims and perpetrators beyond the use of masculine pronouns for the perpetrators and feminine pronouns for the victims. In addition, although the lyrics do not specifically address racial violence, the song's title (which draws from Walt Whitman's anti-slavery poem "I Sing the Body Electric") and reference to Delia Green both suggest an orientation toward racial justice.[9] As a result, the song is broadly applicable to multiple forms of violence, from intimate partner abuse to police brutality to hate crimes.

Because the lack of lyrical detail might seem to give "The Body Electric" less political precision than (say) Nazario's timely reports on a migrant crisis, Segarra has been deliberate about how they perform and describe the song. Specifically, they actively work to preempt what Richie describes as "the everywoman analysis" or an understanding of gender violence as something that potentially affects every (or any) woman. Richie explains that the everywoman concept has "helped to foster an analysis of women's vulnerability as profound and persistent rather than particular to any racial-ethnic community, socioeconomic position, religious group, or station in life" (2012, 90) and has thereby "led to the erasure from the dominant view of the victimization of lesbians, women of color in low-income communities, and other marginalized groups" (91). Segarra insists that "The Body Electric" addresses not violence in general but racialized heteropatriarchal violence in particular. After performing the song on *The Late Show with David Letterman* in June 2014, for instance, Segarra posted an image from the performance to Instagram with a caption that underscored an intersectional analysis of gender violence. Unfortunately, they have since deleted the post, so I am unable to quote it directly, but while researching this chapter I was able to find interviews that offer a similar analysis as the one I recall from Instagram.[10] For instance, Segarra told Powers (2014b): "The song has taught me there is a true connection between gendered violence and racist violence. There is a weaponization of the body happening right now in America. Our bodies are being turned against us. Black and brown bodies are being portrayed as inherently dangerous. . . . It is the same evil idea that leads us to blame women for attacks by their abusers."

Segarra also emphasizes this interpretation in live performances. I saw Hurray for the Riff Raff perform twice when they toured in support of *Small Town Heroes*, in March 2014 and March 2015 (both times in Austin, Texas). The first performance, a sxsw showcase sponsored by a vodka distributor and a corporate bank, at which each member of the audience received free drink tickets, T-shirts, and other swag, did not include the song in its brief set. This was my first time seeing the group live and my first time attending the sxsw music festival; I was at once overwhelmed by the drunken crowd, disappointed that "The Body Electric" was not included in the set, and relieved not to hear a song that fills me with such strong emotions in that raucous environment. The next year, I saw Hurray for the Riff Raff open for civil rights icon Mavis Staples at the Paramount Theater and further appreciated the song's omission from the SXSW set after I saw how Segarra framed the song in this new context. For this performance, most of the group cleared the stage, leaving just Segarra and their longtime collaborator, the fiddler Yosi Perlstein, onstage; the break with the rest of the set gave Segarra the opportunity to introduce the song and its anti-violence message before performing a stripped-down version. Featuring only Perlstein's fiddle and Segarra's haunting voice, this rendition was note-worthy not only for its aesthetic sparseness but also because of the way it highlighted the vulnerable embodiment of a femme of color (Segarra) and a white-presenting transman (Perlstein).

The video for "The Body Electric" further emphasizes an intersectional engagement with violence through visual references to the Black Lives Matter movement and the movement for trans liberation.[11] The video prominently features two Black women: the transgender bounce rapper Katey Red (who poses as Venus in a queer response to Sandro Botticelli's *The Birth of Venus*) and a woman cradling a baby blanket filled with bullet casings, an allusion to Sybrina Fulton, the mother of Trayvon Martin and an outspoken critic of police violence and racial profiling.[12] It is important to note that although the video was directed by Joshua Shoemaker, Segarra was on set through-out its production and was one of the people standing behind the camera throwing the daisies that gently fall around Katey Red in the Botticelli sequence (Fensterstock 2014). Like the lyrics to "The Body Electric," the images of Katey Red and the Black mother figure avoid depicting graphic violence but nonetheless respond to it: by featuring a Black transwoman in the role of Venus, the video imbues her body with the cultural significance of a revered work of art, and by depicting spent bullet casings rising to form the shape of a baby in a woman's arms, the video appeals to viewers to reverse the cultural forces of racialized violence. These images thus affirm the lives of people who—because of the racialization and gendering of their bodies—are uniquely vulnerable to violence.

Both Segarra and Nazario address the intersection between domestic and community or state-sanctioned violence, with Nazario focusing on how gang violence and state neglect foment domestic violence in Central America and Segarra focusing on how racialized gender norms in the United States contribute to relationship violence, police violence, and anti-trans violence. However, whereas Nazario names, describes, and explains the violence directly, Segarra takes a more indirect approach, using their lyrics and performances to affirm the value of lives lost rather than to explicitly narrate the acts of violence. There is certainly a risk in Segarra's approach: the simplicity of their lyrics requires a listener attentive to the social structures they critique because the connections that are clearly drawn in Nazario's work are not as readily apparent. As my analysis makes clear, an appreciation of the political message of "The Body Electric" is not available from simply reading its lyrics; in my case, interpreting the song has required attending Hurray for the Riff Raff shows, seeking out videos online, and following Segarra closely on social media, in addition to playing the song constantly. However, Segarra's emphasis on the lives of victims—the reverent portrayal of Katey Red in the video, the simple but resonant statement in the lyrics that "my girl, we gotta stop it somehow"—also offers a protest that is foreclosed in Nazario's work.

Manuel Muñoz: Imagining Community Accountability

Sexual violence and intimate partner abuse are central themes in the work of Chicano gay writer Manuel Muñoz, with all of his published books to date including some examination of these themes, from stories like "Monkey, Sí" in his 2003 debut short story collection *Zigzagger* to the 2011 novel *What You See in the Dark* (which depicts the murder of a young Mexican American woman by her white male lover). Moreover, as Ralph E. Rodriguez (2018) demonstrates in his beautiful analysis of "Monkey, Sí," Muñoz as a writer is concerned not only with heteropatriarchal violence itself but also with its representation—that is, with the aesthetic choices that render such violence legible and that elicit particular emotional responses. Muñoz's concern with the representation of violence has prompted me to place his work in conversation with anti-violence activists working to develop a framework for responding to violence called *community accountability*. As Ching-In Chen, Jai Dulani, and Leah Lakshmi Piepzna-Samarasinha define it, community accountability entails "any strategy to address violence, abuse or harm that creates safety, justice, reparations, and healing, without relying on police, prisons, childhood protective services, or any other state systems" (2016, xxiii). While the quest to address racialized gender violence outside of state systems might seem idealistic, Chen, Dulani, and Piepzna-Samarasinha are forthright about its challenges: "Community accountability strategies depend on something both potentially more accessible and more complicated: the communities surrounding the person who was harmed and the person who caused harm" (2016, xxiii). Muñoz similarly refuses the idealism that can attach to the word *community*, depicting not just acts of dating and sexual violence but the communities that tolerate it. I argue, therefore, that by exploring what it takes—both ethically and aesthetically—to make violence publicly recognizable within a community structured to conceal it, Muñoz contributes to efforts to explore the possibilities and pitfalls of responding to violence without recourse to the state.

Here I examine two linked stories from Muñoz's second book, the 2007 collection *The Faith Healer of Olive Avenue*: "The Heart Finds Its Own Conclusion" and "The Comeuppance of Lupe Rivera." Both focus on the same two young adults in a small town in California's Central Valley. Cousins Sergio and Cecilia are raised as siblings by the conservative Tío Nico and Tía Sara, separated in childhood when Tía Sara leaves Tío Nico and takes Sergio to Bakersfield, and reunited after Sergio leaves an abusive boyfriend in Bakersfield to move back in with Tío Nico and Cecilia. "The Heart Finds Its Own Conclusion" is narrated in the third person from the perspective of Cecilia, describing an evening when she drives to the bus station in Fresno after receiving a frantic telephone call from Sergio in Bakersfield and encounters a man waiting for him; when the bus arrives, the man forces Sergio into his car and drives away. "The Comeuppance of Lupe Rivera" takes place later, after Sergio has separated from his violent lover, left Bakersfield, and moved back in with Tío Nico and Cecilia; it is narrated in the first person by Sergio, who witnesses an attack on the lover of his neighbor, Lupe Rivera. As it turns out, Lupe's lover is a married man, and his attacker is the brother of the lover's wife. The incident prompts Sergio to meditate on how his community responds differently to the violence unfolding in Lupe's front yard and that occurring in his relationships. Both stories address how community norms governing the expression of gender and sexuality—and the devaluation of women and queers—allow violence to flourish.

Ernesto Javier Martínez observes a technique employed in all of Muñoz's published work, in which the author focalizes events through the perspective of a character who does not directly experience them. Focusing on stories about queer lives told by characters who are not themselves queer, Martínez calls this technique *shifting the site of queer enunciation* and argues that it produces "a deeper understanding of the intersubjective and social contexts in which queer subjects come into being" (2013, 113). In "The Heart Finds

Its Own Conclusion" and "The Comeuppance of Lupe Rivera," however, what we see is a shifting of the site at which domestic violence is enunciated. The effects of this shift are to reveal not only the intersubjective and social contexts that permit violence in intimate relationships but also the role of communities in normalizing or challenging such violence. By shifting the site at which heteropatriarchal violence is enunciated, Muñoz treats the violence as a community responsibility.

"The Heart Finds Its Own Conclusion" (2007) begins with Cecilia waiting in the parking lot of the Fresno bus station for Sergio and remembering a movie she saw as a child with Tío Nico and Tía Sara, a movie featuring "a woman with long black hair, flipped high in front, a woman wearing just pink panties low on the hip" (47), and how "Tía Sara had covered her eyes, tsk-tsked between her teeth" (48). Cecilia recalls the film because she saw it in a movie theater in Fresno located near the bus station, but as the events of the story unfold, it becomes clear not only that watching this movie as a child affects Cecilia's perception of the violence experienced by Sergio but also that, more generally, the stories about gender violence consumed within a community play a role in its response. As the man shoves Sergio into the passenger seat of his car, Cecilia is immobilized:

> The passengers around Cecilia stared at her indecision. The women with children rushed to get their luggage, looking impatiently for their rides, and Cecilia knew what they were thinking. The escalation of arguments, the return of that man, maybe a gun and shots being fired. Hadn't they all seen stories like that? Hadn't they all witnessed what men could do when love was denied? Hadn't they all recognized a man's way of loving, of loving what he could not have? The men from the bus began to walk away, uninterested, and Cecilia silently cursed them through her tears, cursed how ineffectual they were, how their bravado was held in reserve when it really mattered. (65–66)

The bus driver, attempting to comfort Cecilia after she watches the man drive away with her cousin, blames Sergio: "People used to be a lot more civilized. People never acted like this" (66). This prompts Cecilia to remember how she also cried in the movie theater, witnessing the woman's violent end: "As she was bent over the sink, breasts dangling, the backs of her thighs stretched in full view, the men in the theater cheered louder: '¡Eso! ¡Right there! ¡Eso!' The two thugs had begun drowning the woman wearing the pink panties, and that was when Cecilia had rushed from her seat and bolted down the lobby" (68). Both the movie and the night at the bus station find Cecilia devastated by the lack of public support for targets of violence—the woman in the pink panties and her cousin Sergio.

In "The Comeuppance of Lupe Rivera" (2007), Sergio is in Tío Nico's yard checking out "Lupe's latest" (183) when the brother-in-law of her lover shows up:

> I shut off the water hose, and Tío Nico came outside and stood on the lawn, the neighborhood slowly gathering into itself as it did through every argument, through the rare house fires, through the fistfights, the car-bashings from angry ex-wives, the drunkenness of early evening Saturdays, the beating of someone's mother and the shattering windows, the guns flaunted and then desperately coaxed away. The neighborhood inched out of their houses, hands on hips, eyes shaded against sundown, some of the men already easing into the street with order in mind, the younger boys lurking behind them like they knew a rite of passage was theirs for the taking. (187)

Later, Cecilia comes to tell Sergio that Lupe has moved to Los Angeles, and Sergio begins to cry. Although he doesn't tell Cecilia the reason for his tears, he states: "I discovered something that made my heart weight down some. I realized suddenly that, during the times my ex-boyfriends had driven up to Tío Nico's house with their unfamiliar cars and their loud banging and their threats, the street had been empty. No one had come to see about the car still shuddering outside of Tío Nico's house; no one had even come to check to see if Tío Nico was okay" (191–92). Like Cecilia in the earlier story, he cries out of anger that violence in his own relationships is ignored and denied, that he cannot rely on community protection or support, that his own experience will foster no one's rite of passage.

The tears that end both stories—Cecilia's in "The Heart Finds Its Own Conclusion" and Sergio's in "The Comeuppance of Lupe Rivera"—give them a parallel structure. In "The Heart Finds Its Own Conclusion," Cecilia leaves the bus station parking lot knowing that she will soon cry with Tío Nico and remembering how she had cried in the movie theater with Tía Sara. Sergio's tears, meanwhile, are preceded by a moment when Tío Nico finds him looking at the newspaper article about the incident in front of Lupe's home, accompanied by a photo of Lupe's lover crying, and proclaims dismissively: "When grown men cry, . . . it's usually for themselves" (189). In one sense, both Cecilia and Sergio cry for themselves, out of awareness of the ways in which the violence directed at feminine and queer bodies is disregarded and ignored. Martínez writes that crucial "information is conveyed about the sociality of queerness when queer experience is narrated . . . from a narrative voice outside of the experienced events" (2012, 116); this strategy offers "a sense of the diversity of people experiencing queerness, giving us access to the many ways queerness is being conceptualized by people situated differently in relation to it" (116). Likewise, in these two stories, Cecilia and Sergio are situated differently in relation to heteropatriarchal violence but nonetheless recognize themselves and each other as (potential and actual) targets of it. In crying for themselves, Sergio and Cecilia assert the value of their own devalued (feminine/queer, racialized) bodies. More importantly, the tears of Sergio and Cecilia mark the relations of care between them that counter such violence—the nascent beginnings of community accountability. Cecilia recognizes how community norms allow violence to flourish; Sergio, in comparing his experiences to the scene in Lupe Rivera's yard, critiques the way the violence in his relationship is treated as a private, rather than community, concern. In this regard, then, the care Cecilia shows for Sergio, the connections that the cousins recognize between the different forms of violence they endure, have the potential to shift larger structures of violence. It is, to borrow the words of Chen, Dulani, and Piepzna-Samarasinha, a step toward "the radical work of healing—our hearts, our bodies, our families and communities" (2016, xxxv).

Segarra and Muñoz present insights about heteropatriarchal violence not only through the content of their work but through form. In "The Body Electric," the relationship between racial violence and gender violence is not directly highlighted in the lyrics but is made explicit through the use of the murder ballad tradition and through Segarra's performances. In Muñoz's stories, insight about the role of community in fomenting or preventing relationship violence is conveyed not only through the events of the two stories but through the distribution of narrative voice, which highlights Cecilia's role as witness to the violence that Sergio experiences. I emphasize this aspect of both artists' work because it enables me now to directly address a secondary argument of this chapter: that it is not only the texts themselves, but the interpretations of them, that enable their public health interventions. As Paula M. L. Moya points out, an aesthetic object is not simply "a straightforward or ahistorical piece of evidence" (2016, 31); rather, it is in the process of textual analysis that we come to interrogate "the ideas and practices that reflect, promote, and contest the pervasive sociocultural ideals of the world(s) with which the work engages" (36). In other words, it is not merely the act of reading, listening, or watching that enables a work of art to make an intervention but also the act of developing frameworks of interpretation that link the texts back to the reader's social context.

Rigoberto González: Refusing Empathy

I emphasize the importance of interpretation as I turn to the work of Rigoberto González, arguing that his 2006 memoir *Butterfly Boy: Memories of Chicano Mariposa* resists "commonsense" ideas about heteropatriarchal violence that establish which victims deserve support and empathy (and, thus, by extension, which victims do not).[13] Like Piepzna-Samarasinha, who begins their memoir of intergenerational abuse survival by alerting the reader that "my therapist is not a major character in it, and the therapy sessions, court dates, and talking with nice policemen, ditto" (2015, 15), González offers a memoir of intergenerational abuse that departs significantly from the conventions of the genre—and, more specifically, from the demands of the genre to represent an abuse survivor who elicits empathy in the reader. In her famous critique of nineteenth-century abolitionist discourse, Hartman examines "the repressive effects of empathy," which presents the vulnerable and suffering body as "a vessel for the uses, thoughts, and feelings of others" (1997, 19). The influence of Hartman's critical skepticism toward empathy is evident not only in African American studies but extends across a wide range of fields, including two of particular interest to me here: feminist memoir studies and the health humanities. In this section, I explore how the refusal to cultivate an empathetic reader in *Butterfly Boy* advances a critical framework for understanding and responding to violence.

Butterfly Boy follows Rigoberto through the summer of 1990, as he leaves his abusive lover in the United States (Riverside, California), accompanies his father on a bus journey to his father's birthplace in Mexico (Zacapu, Michoacán), then returns to Riverside for an encounter with his lover that ends the book. Interspersed with stories from the summer of 1990 are memories from Rigoberto's childhood and "ghost whispers," the stories that he tells his lover about his life. The back-and-forth narrative structure of the memoir reflects the migration patterns of the monarch butterfly alluded to in the memoir's title, which also links together two of its major themes: the González family's four generations of border crossings, and Rigoberto's cycles of leaving and returning to his lover, a pattern often seen in abusive relationships.

Because representations of domestic abuse often end triumphantly with the victim leaving the abuser, readers are primed to expect such a story in *Butterfly Boy*, and the first chapter seems to set up such a narrative. The book begins the morning after a particularly violent argument between Rigoberto and his lover: "This break-up isn't following the pattern of all the other ones we've had. There's no pleading after the fight and the fuck" (6). As he closes the door to his lover's apartment, Rigoberto tests the knob: "Yes, I've definitely locked myself out" (7). Despite these early hints at a permanent separation, Rigoberto's trip to Michoacán is punctuated by erotic thoughts of his lover and by ghost whispers addressing the lover with the endearment "querido." At the end of the book, when he returns to Riverside, Rigoberto immediately calls his lover: "Soon we are eating in the same restaurants, ordering the same dishes, drinking the same wines" (198). The book ends with him leaving his lover's apartment after another brutal fight, followed by a final ghost whisper. While it is tempting (again) to read this exit as the end of the relationship, the fact that the memoir begins with a similar scene makes it difficult to assert with any certainty that the cycle is, in fact, over.

If one of Muñoz's signature styles is his unusual focalization, one of González's is maintaining emotional distance between his characters and his readers. Reviews and critical studies of his work frequently address this distance, sometimes with more than a hint of disparagement. In a review of González's earlier novel *Crossing Vines* for *Library Journal*, Lawrence Olszewski determines that the novel "fails to show us characters with strong individual identities" so that "the reader can't care about their plight"; he ultimately recommends the book "only for libraries serving Hispanic communities" (2003, 91). Nancy Kang's review of *Butterfly Boy* for *Callaloo* is more sympathetic, but she also confesses frustration: "The risk-taking and the drama prove, at times, emotionally exhausting" (2014, 752). Although Olszewski and Kang critique the way González seems to discourage readers from emotional investment in his characters, literary critic Colleen Gleeson Eils reads this distance as a deliberate narrative strategy; she argues that by limiting "readers' access to characters' lives," González challenges "the role of native informant so often expected of nonwhite and indigenous authors by US audiences, instead creating spaces of narrative privacy" (2017, 31). Eils focuses her argument on *Crossing Vines*, but it can also be adapted to *Butterfly Boy*, where González refuses the narrative structure (a clean break from an abusive lover) typically used to spark readers' empathy; by limiting readers' emotional access, he calls into question the terms by which survivors of relationship violence are deemed worthy of empathy. I argue that the "spaces of narrative privacy" that González creates in *Butterfly Boy* force readers to confront their expectations of both the memoir form and the actions of abuse survivors.

It is important to note that although literary representations of intimate partner violence often conclude with the end of the violent relationship, real-life stories are often much more complicated. Ending the relationship does not always end the abuse, and victims of relationship violence often return to their violent lovers over and over, for numerous reasons.[14] Kang's review of *Butterfly Boy* reflects the frustration that can attend to the experience of supporting a person in a violent relationship: "Readers hope the memoirist will finally quit his Svengali, but even after being publicly humiliated, beaten, and raped, the writer withholds any promise of resolution" (2014, 752). The unresolved ending leads Kang to describe *Butterfly Boy* as "disappointing" (753); she laments that although "optimistic readers might seek the promise of supportive friends or a better romantic partner for the memoirist, no such comfort is forthcoming" (753). Kang's disappointment in the narrative arc of *Butterfly Boy* is often shared by those witnessing a loved one in a violent relationship. Resources for advocates note the importance of respecting survivors' decisions not to leave; as the National Domestic Violence Hotline (n.d.), for instance, warns on its "Help for Friends and Family" page: "There are many reasons why victims stay in abusive relationships. They may leave and return to the relationship many times. Do not criticize their decisions or try to guilt them. They will need your support even more during those times." This is advice, however, that I have often found extraordinarily difficult to take; my research on the topic and my extensive conversations with friends who have also witnessed such abuse suggests that I am not alone. I wonder, therefore, if it is so hard to take this advice in part because people who have not directly faced relationship violence often access the experience through narratives that, by framing the end of the relationship as a triumphant conclusion, occlude the complications of ending an abusive relationship.

González does not offer the reasons typically mobilized to explain the choice to stay in a violent relationship: Rigoberto does not share a home or have children with his lover; he is not dependent on his lover for basic sustenance; he does not appear to fear his lover's retaliation. This may make it even harder to understand why he returns. Kang perceptively cites passages indicating that "because of pervasive silences around same-sex coupling . . . , he was largely confused" (2014, 753). Perhaps more important, however, is the fact that Rigoberto, like many people experiencing relationship violence, enjoys aspects of his relationship. His lover gives him gifts: "The watch keeping time on my right wrist is a gift from him. The black leather band and convex glass over the pearl-colored face make me feel elegant" (González 2006, 4). His lover is attractive: "His strong arms . . . they're the feature of his that I admire the most. They're the parts of his body I reach for when I wake up in the middle of the night and I want to remind myself that my lover, all muscle and strength, is still in bed beside me" (7). His lover takes him to restaurants where he learns "about wines, Italian desserts, and condiments so tasty and exotic they're like portholes into other parts of the world" (36). For a reader who believes that it is "common sense" for an abuse survivor to leave a relationship unless there is a compelling reason to stay, these reasons may feel inadequate.

However, I argue that it is precisely *because* Rigoberto's return to his lover risks "exhausting" and "disappointing" the reader (to use Kang's words), subverting the "commonsense" strategies that texts often deploy in order to cultivate readerly empathy, that *Butterfly Boy* offers an important contribution to understandings of relationship violence. By elaborating how abolitionist narratives used empathy to position Blackness as "the imaginative surface upon which the master and the nation came to understand themselves" (1997, 7), Hartman reminds us that the function of empathy is often to direct audiences back to *their own* ethical and aesthetic frameworks, not those of the objects of their empathy. For this reason, health humanities scholar Rebecca Garden asserts that empathy "often develops in tandem with judgement and with the evaluation of worthiness" (2013, 447–48), while memoir scholar Leigh Gilmore notes that when a survivor's story does not align with a reader's value system, empathy may fail—and "when empathy fails, doubt and discrediting emerge" (2017, 130).[15] By refusing to court readers' empathy and instead provoking an analysis of what Hartman calls "the significance of opacity" (1997, 36), *Butterfly Boy* draws attention to the criteria by which readers will evaluate Rigoberto's "worthiness" for empathy.

Like the scholars just cited, I advocate an approach to literary studies that fosters both critical and ethical awareness; I also advocate attention to texts' formal and generic features. Here I return to a point from my summary of the memoir's plot: the text's allusions to the migration patterns of the monarch butterfly structure both its narrative (Rigoberto's journey from Riverside to Zacapu and back) and its two major themes (labor migrations between Michoacán and California and the cycles of leaving and returning common in abusive relationships).[16] The butterfly—and particularly the monarch—is an important symbol of both Latinx queer masculinity and of migrant rights activists, and as Daniel Enrique Pérez (2014) notes, it is a symbol that recurs across many of González's published works.[17] In *Butterfly Boy*, access to Rigoberto's story in an emotional register not dependent on empathy becomes available through attention to its formal dimensions, particularly its symbolic deployment of the monarch butterfly to represent both multigenerational migration and intimate partner violence.

González introduces the butterfly on the first page, revealing that Rigoberto and his lover refer to the bruises left on Rigoberto's skin during sex as *butterflies*:

> "I just gave you another butterfly," he says. And I know then we are meant for each other because his gift matches my fantasy tattoo: I want a path of monarchs spiraling out of the base of my back and spreading open like a tornado, the insects growing in size as they flutter up toward my shoulders. Monarchs, I tell him, remind me of home and of my family.
> "But I thought you hated home and your family," he says.
> "But I love them too," I say. (2006, 3)

Like the family Rigoberto loves and hates, the bruises evoke powerfully ambivalent emotions. He calls them "art" (3) and associates them with "sheet-twisting nights of sex and sweat" (3), but he also describes them as painful and reveals that they are not exactly consensual: "I never ask my lover for butterflies and neither does he seek permission" (4). The butterfly resurfaces, linked to labor migrations, when Rigoberto introduces his family history:

> I was born into a culture of work. Since the age of the Bracero Program of the 1940s, the state of Michoacán has been the number one exporter of Mexican farm labor to the United States. It is not out of the ordinary to witness entire communities of farmworkers migrate back and forth between the two countries—an echo of the region's famous monarch butterflies who do the same for survival, their spectacular flights across the continent retraced generations later through genetic memory. When we descended on Thermal [a town in California's Coachella Valley], los González were no strangers to dramatic change. We had been moving north and south for four generations, which explains why my great-grandfather and father were Mexican-born citizens, while my grandfather and I were U.S.-born citizens. (55)

The monarch butterfly might be beautiful, but it is clear from these passages that it is not an unequivocally positive symbol for González; it evokes physical and sexual abuse, physically exhausting labor, and physical and economic dispossession. Pérez observes that *mariposas* (both butterflies and queer men) are "resilient in harsh, foreign, and homophobic environments" (2014, 103); González reinforces this point by emphasizing the harsh conditions that Rigoberto survives. Indeed, González's invocation of the four generations of his family who have crossed the US-Mexico border for work alludes to a little-known and disconcerting fact about the monarch butterfly: no single insect ever carries out the full migration cycle; rather, butterflies continually die along the way, and completing the route requires four generations. The butterfly, then, is linked not only to beauty and survival but also to death. Understanding the complexity of the butterfly symbol for González, then, is crucial to understanding the complexity of its emotional registers, particularly the profound ambivalence with which Rigoberto approaches his family, his personal history, and his relationship. Rigoberto's relationship with his lover cannot be understood without understanding the history of unequal relations between the United States and Mexico that have fostered the four generations of economic, social, familial, and romantic precarity that Rigoberto inherits.

It may seem ironic that *Butterfly Boy*—a work of creative nonfiction—requires so much more interpretive labor from readers than many fictional representations of intimate partner abuse; common sense would have it that nonfictional events are straightforward, requiring no interpretation (although scholars in memoir and nonfiction studies would certainly point out the fallacy of this assumption). Because it lacks the straightforward ending that a fictional plot can easily achieve—the clean break with the violent lover—the text forces its readers to confront their expectations not only about what a portrayal of relationship violence should accomplish but also about how a survivor should act. By straining the reader's capacity for empathy and refusing to depict a clean break, González demands that his reader engage with the text at multiple levels: plot, historical and social context, form. In doing so, he raises questions about the social structures and aesthetic modes that produce or foreclose empathy for survivors of domestic abuse.

Angie Cruz: Healing without a Cure

My final case study for this chapter is a novel that depicts intimate partner violence in a situation of extreme power imbalance. In interviews, at readings, and in her biography on the jacket, author Angie Cruz identifies *Dominicana*

(2019) as a biographical novel based on her mother's life.[18] *Dominicana* is the story of Ana Canción, a fifteen-year-old girl from the Dominican countryside forced into an arranged marriage with Juan Ruiz, a man in his thirties who lives in New York City, to facilitate her family's immigration to the United States. The novel is divided into five parts that depict Ana's adolescence in Los Guayacanes, Dominican Republic, including Juan's negotiations with Ana's family (Part I); Ana's move to New York City and Juan's physical and sexual abuse of her (Part II); Ana's pregnancy (Part III); Juan's return to the Dominican Republic to secure family assets before the 1965 US invasion and the beginning of Ana's affair with Juan's younger brother César (Part IV); and finally Juan's return, the birth of Ana's child, and the arrival of her mother and brother to New York City (Part V). Addressing the intersection of migration and domestic abuse, *Dominicana* examines the possibilities for imagining radical health after gender violence when the social conditions that gave rise to the violence remain intact.

Much of the novel takes place in a small apartment overlooking the Audubon Ballroom, located in the same building in Washington Heights where Cruz herself grew up; it is the site of both Ana's confinement and her acts of resistance, like cooking a pigeon for Juan's dinner (in a failed attempt to give him food poisoning), finding ways to earn money without his knowledge, and eventually initiating a sexual relationship with his younger brother. While the novel follows some aspects of Cruz's family history, it also includes an important departure, as Cruz reveals in an interview: "My family was in NYC in the '70s, but for *Dominicana*, I was interested in writing about 1965. That was the year the U.S. occupied D.R. It was the year Malcolm X was shot across from the building I grew up in [in Washington Heights]. I wanted to bring all these historical moments together and show how, even if they're different stories and movements, they're all interconnected" (Bansinath 2019). This move is consistent with a political gesture visible in much Dominican diasporic fiction, which, as Lorgia García-Peña observes, "places the Dominican experience within US history by insisting on the long and unequal relationship between the two nations" while also historicizing "dominicanidad from the margins, letting other voices speak" (2016, 84). Building on García-Peña's point, I argue that Cruz's decision to set the novel in 1965 is critical not only to its transnational racial politics but also to its depiction of intimate partner violence.

Dominicana unfolds in short, episodic chapters. In an economical four pages, its first chapter succinctly establishes the unequal relationship between Ana and Juan. The novel begins: "The first time Juan Ruiz proposes,

I'm eleven years old, skinny and flat-chested" (Cruz 2019, 3), immediately invoking the age difference that will reinforce Juan's individual power over Ana. From this opening, Cruz moves quickly to the socioeconomic differences between the Ruiz and Canción families, which are themselves linked to the geopolitical relationship between the Dominican Republic and the United States. Juan and his brothers, Ana explains, show up every other weekend "all the way from La Capital to serenade the good country girls who're eligible for marriage" (3) and "clang on Papá's colmado's bell as if they're herding cows" (3). Why are they able to behave in this way? "Everyone knows who the Ruiz brothers are because they travel to and from New York, returning with pockets full of dollars" (4). The Canción family, by contrast, struggles to eke out a living in the political instability that follows the assassination of the dictator Rafael Trujillo: "There'd been some chicken stealing, and our store had been robbed twice in the past year. So we keep everything under lock and key, especially after Trujillo was shot dead. . . . But Trujillo didn't go in peace. La Capital is in chaos. A tremendous mess" (3). From the very beginning, then, Ana's individual disempowerment is a microcosm of the hemispheric dominance of the United States.

Ana's mother also plays a key role in her abuse, as she is the one who facilitates Ana's marriage to Juan. The novel does not delve into Ana's mother's personal history but does make clear both the racial discrimination she experiences within the Dominican Republic and its ultimate implications for her green-eyed daughter: "From birth, Mamá says, my eyes were a winning lottery ticket, inherited from my grandfather from El Cibao. She talks proudly about Papá's family, even though they'd cut us all off after Mamá married Papá thinking he would take her far away from Los Guayacanes. Ever hopeful, Mamá had ignored the warnings that those people don't mix with blacks" (11). Later, once Ana is trapped in New York City with Juan, her fantasies of leaving are tempered with the knowledge of how her mother will respond: "If I leave Juan and return home, this is the way Mamá will prepare for my arrival. On the table she'll have laid out a plastic slipper, my father's leather belt, a sack of uncooked rice, a ream from a tree, the fly swatter, and a wire hanger. . . . She'll make me choose from the instruments" (100). Cruz is unsparing in both her depiction of Ana's mother and her depiction of the poverty (exacerbated by racial discrimination) that Ana's mother is seeking to mitigate: "Mamá points at some barefooted boys carrying baskets of bags filled with peanuts and peeled oranges. Do you know what your brother Yohnny is doing every day while you and Lenny spend your mornings at school?" (26). These passages serve not to exonerate Ana's mother but rather to highlight the impossibility of the situation that the entire Canción family is in and the layers of gendered and racialized oppression that Ana bears.

Once in New York City, Ana observes how the white supremacist logics that facilitated her marriage to Juan operate within the context of the United States. This education begins when she witnesses the assassination of Malcolm X through the window of her apartment: "Before I heard the gunshots I noticed the army of bow-tie-wearing black men enter the Audubon Ballroom, their families trailing behind them. Usually the cops hover nearby, but today there are none around" (76). At first, she is interested in the events only because she sees her neighborhood on television: "Behind the dead man on the stretcher onscreen is the dental-supplies store and the small park where Juan and I sometimes sit on a bench and share an ice cream. There it is, our Broadway, making the news! The 168th Street subway entrance, the emergency room sign. Our building!" (78). As she follows the story, however, Ana demonstrates a growing sensitivity to Juan's racism—"Juan says *those blacks* as if he's skinning a goat" (86)—and to the demonstrations she sees from her window: "People march with flowers, photos of Malcolm X, and poster boards" (113). As Raphael Dalleo and Elena Machado Sáez have stated about earlier work by Cruz, the novel moves toward "a transformative recontextualization of the U.S. Latino/a experience within the larger framework of the hemisphere" to highlight "the public and personal histories of marginality and exploitation that fragment and connect Las Américas" (2007, 101). Ana's fascination with Malcolm X thus represents not only the logics of white supremacy at work in both the United States and the Dominican Republic but also her own growing critique of these logics, as she begins to develop an awareness of herself and her circumstances as imbricated within a larger history. This is especially clear when she differentiates her own perception of historical events like Malcolm X's assassination from Juan's perception.

The novel oscillates between presenting Ana as subjected to history and as an agent within her own history. For instance, it is useful to consider the first scene in which Ana experiences violence, the night of her marriage to Juan and the morning before leaving for New York, in a hotel room in Santo Domingo. Juan undresses Ana, she resists having sex with him, and he coaxes her first gently and then forcefully. Cruz avoids giving traumatizing details of the rape, depicting it through sparse dialogue and spare details:

> He presses his bulge against my back. I cry. He turns me around
> so I face him.

I want to go home. Please.

This is your home. Me and you are a family now. Don't you see.

The crying comes faster and harder. It can't be true. I have a
family. I have a home.

I want to go home, I repeat, my voice smaller, broken. (2019, 46)

Here Ana's trauma is conveyed primarily through the details of the dialogue, the description of her "smaller, broken" voice, and the fact of her tears. The actual rape is contained in one short, evocative sentence: "The pain, short and sharp" (48). Later, after Ana becomes pregnant and goes to a prenatal checkup, the extent of Juan's violence is revealed in the description of her body and the doctor's response: "She notes some bruises on my arm and neck from so many weeks ago—but they take forever to heal" (132); the doctor then gives her "glossy papers" (133) featuring images of "a woman with a busted lip and a black eye filled with panic" (133). In these scenes, Cruz avoids overly graphic descriptions of the violence Ana experiences but also emphasizes her lack of power; the violence seems to happen not to the protagonist of the text but to another body that she merely describes.

The sparse narration of the violence Ana experiences stands in distinct contrast to the moments when Ana takes sexual initiative with partners of her choosing. For instance, the day before her marriage, Ana kisses her school crush, Gabriel: "I kiss him, right on the mouth. . . . Our full lips closed tight like our eyes, they press against each other like soft pillows. My insides spin around as if I'm still in the water. A thread pulls up between my legs, through my heart and up my throat" (30–31). Later, while Juan is in the Dominican Republic, she has sex with his brother César: "His pistol springs up and points at me and for the first time I don't cringe or look away. I stare at it. Grab it. I want it inside of me. . . . I grab him and push him inside me. I don't care if I die right there. I want him to thrust inside of me forever. Let this be our last day. Let us die right here" (265). By emphasizing the description of Ana's consensual encounters, even as she also depicts the effects of Juan's violence, Cruz portrays Ana as sexual agent as well as victim.

Cruz's balance between emphasizing Ana's agency and her victimization is also evident in the novel's title. Although *Dominicana* might seem to refer first and foremost to Ana's national origin and to evoke a kind of everywoman migration story, the Dominicana that surfaces most often in the novel is a doll where Ana hides the money she earns behind Juan's back from sewing and cooking. The faceless doll, one of the Dominican

Republican's best-known handicrafts, is a wedding gift from Juan: "I place the ceramic doll Juan bought me at the airport in Santo Domingo on the table. She wears a blue dress and a yellow sash around her waist. My sweet, hollow Dominicana will keep all my secrets: she has no eyes, no lips, no mouth" (58). Like Ana, the doll with "no eyes, no lips, no mouth" appears submissive on the surface but guards secrets and money, enabling Ana to make independent preparations for the arrival of her family.

The pacing of the novel speeds up rapidly at the end. While Juan is in the Dominican Republic, Ana and César plan to move to Boston together, only to have their plans interrupted by Juan's news that he is bringing Ana's mother and younger brother to New York City. Choosing her family over César, Ana stays with Juan, whose abuse of her is revealed to Ana's mother when he hits her and causes a postpartum hemorrhage shortly after the birth of her baby: "Finally she understands everything I have sacrificed, everything I have survived for her and for the family" (317).[19] The novel ends uneasily, with Ana, her mother, and her brother still living with Juan in their one-bedroom apartment (now reconfigured: Ana sleeps with her mother and brother, while Juan sleeps in the living room), but Ana imagines a future without him. Despite Ana's optimism, a number of questions remain unanswered: Is it safe for Ana to continue living with Juan, even temporarily? Is it safe for her to leave? Does the presence of her mother and brother make her safer or increase her dependence? With her mother and brother working, has the economic balance in the home shifted so that Juan no longer has control? Does Ana's mother recognize Ana's sacrifices enough to finally protect her? Like González in *Butterfly Boy*, Cruz refuses to resolve her protagonist's situation at the end, reflecting the reality of many domestic abuse survivors for whom separation from an abusive partner can be a long and complicated process. Yet, unlike *Butterfly Boy*, *Dominicana* ends with a surprisingly optimistic tone.

I conclude this section with a consideration of the significance of this optimism. In an interview with fellow Dominican writer Nelly Rosario, published just before she began writing *Dominicana*, Cruz states: "Fiction is one of those last places where the world is bound between these pages, and you can sit with it for awhile and imagine humanity in a completely different way. . . . I don't want to write the war in my next novel. I want to imagine peace" (Cruz and Rosario 2007, 748). Building from Cruz's statement, I suggest that there are important political ramifications to both González's ominous ending and to Cruz's more positive one. González's ending, as I argued, offers a dose of realism that is important for advocates and others seeking to understand the experience of intimate partner abuse, particularly those who don't understand why victims stay with their abusers. At the same time, by ending this chapter with Cruz's novel, I note that equally important is the impulse to (as Cruz puts it) "imagine humanity in a completely different way." How might we begin to imagine different worlds for women like Ana, or for the other characters discussed in this chapter? Crucially, Ana finds no resolution in traditional legal or medical institutions; the brochures about domestic abuse given to her by her doctor accomplish nothing but stoking Juan's rage. Cruz's novel—like the other texts discussed here—suggests that what is ultimately needed is a radical restructuring of the sociopolitical forces that devalue immigrant women like Ana, from US dominance in the hemisphere to everyday instantiations of white supremacy and misogyny. And while this radical restructuring might seem too abstract to imagine, Cruz suggests that it begins with a restructuring of family and community life.

Remedio

There are times when writing flows: words come together on the page and appear to arrange themselves; thoughts cohere effortlessly. This chapter did not offer one of those experiences. It took years to take shape: a scan of my cv tells me that the first conference paper (on Manuel Muñoz) that became this chapter was written in 2015, but it wasn't until late 2019, when I had a fellowship, that I began writing the full analysis I had dreamed of when I wrote that first conference paper. That first draft also took months out of a fellowship year; active writing days would go by with my word count stubbornly unchanged. Even once I finally produced a full draft of this chapter, it never felt finished: this chapter was always the one for which outside readers had the most suggestions and questions. I have, at this point, reached a state where I feel confident in each of the individual close readings contained herein. I think I am saying new and important things about the texts, at least. But about gender violence? The truth is, I've always felt compelled to speak about it but unsure whether I have anything important to say. I've never felt that my own responses to it were adequate, not when it happened to me and not when it happened to my (many) loved ones. Why did it take me so long to recognize that I was in a dangerous situation? Why haven't I ever been able to save people I love?

Despite the difficulty of writing this chapter, it has also been the most important to me. Like Piepzna-Samarasinha, I have always been drawn to stories about domestic violence and frustrated with the solutions offered by many of the available stories. I started writing about Manuel Muñoz before I knew what this book was about. All I knew was that I needed those stories about Sergio and Cecilia, needed the model of their love and loyalty to each other even when they didn't know what to do or how to express it. I needed Cecilia in the parking lot of the bus station, watching her cousin being driven away by his violent lover and not being able to save him but also refusing to give up on him. I needed the messy ending.

"What if some things aren't fixable?" asks Piepzna-Samarasinha (2018, 235). She continues: "I believe in healing and I believe in it happening in ways that are mind-blowing and far beyond what anyone thought possible. But I also wonder, what if some trauma wounds really never will go away—and we might still have great lives?" (235). For Piepzna-Samarasinha, the crucial difference between healing and being cured is that the trauma wounds are still present after healing; the experience and its traces (including the knowledge and the skills that it offers) remain. For me, this is the crux of what I mean by *radical health*. I want to write against a pervasive cultural narrative that a healthy response to violence means a clean break between abused and abuser, means suturing the wounds and erasing the scars, means returning magically to a time "before" the abuse. Although this chapter may seem much less informed by disability studies than the ones that precede it, it is in fact deeply indebted to the work of disability justice activists like Piepzna-Samarasinha and disability studies scholars like Eunjung Kim who problematize the concept of cure, reminding us that "cure is always a multifaceted negotiation, often enabling and disabling at the same time, and may be accompanied by pain, loss, or death" (E. Kim 2017, 7). In particular, one significant loss that ensues from a desire to individually "cure" instantiations of gender violence by simply separating abuser and abused and urging the abused to "move on" is leaving intact the societal infrastructure that facilitated the abuse in the first place.

Radical health after abuse, for me, means reckoning with the larger context that foments abuse—what Piepzna-Samarasinha calls the "the water and the air" (2018, 140) of a society that systemically devalues racialized and feminized people—and also means not asking survivors how they ended up in abusive relationships or why they stayed in them; it means prioritizing interventions that address the sociopolitical context of violence over those focusing on the actions or attributes of the victims. Furthermore, it requires an acknowledgment that although domestic violence is inherently gendered, it is not exclusively so; interventions that account exclusively for gender and not for race, class, immigration status, and other axes of oppression will likewise be ineffective.

But how do we do that? It's absolutely true that there aren't a plethora of models or practical guides out there. Indeed, Chen, Dulani, and Piepzna-Samarasinha—whose coedited volume *The Revolution Starts at Home: Confronting Intimate Violence within Activist Communities* seeks to compile activist resources for confronting violence—describe their own efforts at theorizing community accountability work as still deeply speculative and experimental: "bushwhacking our way through alleyways, back roads, and starlit fields without maps" (2016, xxii). The texts I've discussed here are not a practical guide, per se, but they have offered me inspiration in imagining the world otherwise. As I've noted in the remedios to prior chapters, I believe deeply in the power of art as a social intervention. These texts show us what we need and allow us to begin to think about what it would take to get it. In other words, art must be part of the remedio itself.

4

Mental Health and Migrant Justice

Family Separation and Reimagining Wellness

In May 2018, President Donald Trump made official a strategy his administration had been quietly testing for months, a "zero tolerance" policy to charge migrants with illegal entry and send them into federal detention without their children—*after* they complied with US law by presenting themselves at border checkpoints to request asylum. Thousands of children, some under six months old, were taken from their parents and placed into the custody of the US Department of Health and Human Services with no plan for family reunification (Dickerson 2019; Kates 2018; Kopan 2018). The international outcry was swift and intense, and on June 20, 2018, Trump was forced to sign an executive order ostensibly discontinuing family separations. While the official policy lasted only six weeks, migrant children continued to be taken from their parents (albeit via different legal mechanisms, prompting less outrage) throughout Trump's term in office.[1] More importantly, the psychological damage has lasted much longer—indeed, it is still unfolding, among those reunited as well as among the hundreds (perhaps thousands) of families who remain separated.[2]

Accused of harming children, the Trump administration shifted the blame to migrant parents. In the immediate aftermath of the crisis, Trump's daughter and senior advisor Ivanka Trump sought to characterize asylum seekers as lawbreakers who put their own children in harm's way: "I am the daughter of an immigrant, my mother grew up in communist Czech Republic, but we are a country of laws. She came to this country legally and we have to be very careful about incentivizing behavior that puts children at risk of being trafficked, at risk of entering this country with coyotes or making an incredibly dangerous journey alone" (Klein 2018). A year later, Secretary of Homeland Security Kirstjen Nielsen, who had implemented the zero tolerance policy, reflected in a PBS *NewsHour* interview: "I don't regret enforcing the law" because "not to enforce the law would encourage trafficking, would encourage . . . children to be used as pawns" (Woodruff and Nawaz 2019).[3] She used the word "heartbreaking," not to describe how migrants were treated under her watch, but rather to describe the actions of parents who bring their children on "a terrible, dangerous journey" (Woodruff and Nawaz 2019).

Of course, Trump and his allies are easy targets for a discussion of the psychological harms inflicted by US border enforcement policies, the topic of this chapter. However, the rhetorical move of impugning migrant parents for the maltreatment of children by US officials frequently goes unchallenged (and, in some cases, is even used) by self-proclaimed migrant advocates. For instance, the journalist Sonia Nazario, whose work is discussed in chapter 3, states as a motivation for her best-selling book *Enrique's Journey* the goal of helping Latina mothers to "understand the full consequences of leaving their children behind and make better-informed decisions" (2007, xxv).[4] And a year before Trump's family separations, President Barack Obama rebuked his successor on Facebook for rescinding the Deferred Action for Childhood Arrivals (DACA) order. While defending DACA recipients, Obama (2017) also implicitly vilified their parents, criticizing the move "to expel talented, driven, patriotic young people from the only country they know solely because of the actions of their parents."

The political gains achieved by asserting the virtue of child migrants are not insignificant. Ana Elena Puga and Víctor M. Espinosa explain: "Children are effective political agents precisely because they are perceived to be above or beside the point of politics. Moreover, because their existence heralds the future, their individually suffering bodies can help create social bodies and social policy organized around hopes for a better future" (2020, 237).

Public anguish over the treatment of migrant children forced Trump to end zero tolerance. Public support for DACA prevented Trump from rescinding the Obama-era policy.

And yet the move to secure migrant justice through the figure of the child deserves scrutiny as well. Children constitute such malleable political symbols that it is possible even for those as complicit as Ms. Trump and Secretary Nielsen to purport to act in their interest; no matter how intentional an act of state-sponsored child abuse, it can apparently be cloaked in rhetoric about protecting children.[5] More importantly, as Obama's defense of DACA shows, assertions of the child migrant's innocence risk locating guilt in the migrant parent. Lee Edelman famously argues that the "sacralization of the Child . . . necessitates the sacrifice of the queer" (2004, 28); it might similarly be said that in immigration politics the sacralization of the child migrant (or student, or DREAMer) often seems to necessitate the sacrifice of the parent.[6] Here it is instructive to compare DACA with another Obama-era executive order, Deferred Action for Parents of Americans and Lawful Permanent Residents (DAPA), which would have shielded undocumented parents of US citizens and permanent residents from deportation. Whereas DACA's broad appeal protected it from Trump's assaults, DAPA never went into effect: it was immediately challenged in federal court before being quietly rescinded by Trump when Obama left office. And whereas Trump's successor, President Joe Biden, claims to be making it a priority to preserve and strengthen DACA, efforts to revive DAPA have not materialized as of this writing. Meanwhile, an estimated 5.1 million US citizen children live with at least one undocumented parent who is vulnerable to deportation (Capps, Fix, and Zong 2016), and the fear of parental deportation has dire mental health consequences for children in mixed-status families (Human Impact Partners 2018).

Although migrant parents have been overlooked at best and maligned at worst by politicians and pundits, Latinx expressive culture reassesses their actions and circumstances and, in so doing, expands both the conversation around the wellbeing of child migrants and the political horizons of immigration activism. In the immediate aftermath of Trump's family separation debacle, the writer Reyna Grande (2018) published an editorial in the *New York Times* responding to Ms. Trump's comments about Central American parents: "No parent wants to uproot and risk his or her child's life. Unlike Ms. Trump's mother, my father was an economic migrant, too poor to qualify for even the most basic visa requirements. He was a maintenance worker with a third-grade education, and the only way to give his children a better future was to break the law." Grande thus refuses a logic that would affirm her own innocence at her father's expense. Yet, in other writings, Grande also painfully details her parents' shortcomings and mistakes. Her memoirs depict the physical and emotional abuse she experienced as a child, by relatives in Mexico and by her parents in the United States; her father's violence and alcohol dependence; and her mother's neglect. Even as she vehemently critiques Ms. Trump for "putting the blame on immigrants" (2018), Grande does not idealize her own immigrant parents. Instead, she offers a nuanced portrait of parental figures who both experience and perpetuate trauma—a representation that, I argue in this chapter, offers a more powerful resource for imagining radical mental health than a simple claim to innocence. Like the cultural workers described in previous chapters, who both demand conditions for wellbeing while refusing to stigmatize unwellness, Grande denounces the psychological harms inflicted on her family because of US border enforcement policy while also working to destigmatize the mental health consequences of those harms.

Family separation and its psychic toll is a prominent concern for many Latinx cultural workers. Although the issue became a national flash point during the Trump years, US border enforcement has separated families since the late 1800s, when its first immigration restrictions took effect. According to the literary critic Marta Caminero-Santangelo (2016), undocumented migrations—including the family separations that often result—have become an increasingly prominent theme in Latinx literature since 1994, when President Bill Clinton launched the border enforcement initiative known as Operation Gatekeeper.[7] In this chapter, I examine the work of four Latinx writers separated from their parents as children—Grande, Junot Díaz, Javier Zamora, and Karla Cornejo Villavicencio—to elaborate how each depicts family separation and its mental health effects. Although the texts examined here address geopolitical contexts that precede the Trump-era crisis, they offer necessary insights on its long-term effects. The writers examined in this chapter depict US immigration policy as a threat to the mental and physical health of *both* migrant children *and* their parents. I begin with texts that address pre-Gatekeeper migrations and move toward more contemporary contexts; as I do so, I also move from more straightforward depictions of migration (memoir, narrative fiction) to more experimental ones (poetry, creative nonfiction). Read together, these works offer an opportunity to consider how the notion of radical health I have developed throughout this book extends to literary engagements with mental health.

In the work of Grande, Díaz, Zamora, and Cornejo, migrant parents are often as traumatized as their children—and, indeed, their children often suffer because of their trauma. The texts I have chosen to analyze in this chapter, then, take political risks as well as aesthetic ones. As a result, they offer an opportunity to engage with recent scholarship in Latinx studies reassessing inspirational aesthetics, as well as with mad studies scholarship treating trauma and other forms of psychiatric debilitation "not only as medical conditions but also as historical formations that have justified all manner of ill-treatment and disenfranchisement—even as they have also formed the basis for political identities, social movements, and cultural practices of resistance" (Aho, Ben-Moshe, and Hilton 2017, 293). For instance, Leticia Alvarado highlights representations that "cohere their aesthetic gestures around negative affects—uncertainty, disgust, unbelonging—capturing what lies far outside mainstream, inspirational Latino-centered social justice struggles" (2018, 4). Although building a political movement based around sympathetic figures—"kids who study in our schools, young adults who are starting careers, patriots who pledge allegiance to our flag," as Obama (2017) put it—might seem efficacious, such a movement will ultimately exclude many it purports to defend. By representing migrant families in their full complexity, the authors discussed here offer what La Marr Jurelle Bruce calls a "mad methodology [that] primes us to extend *radical compassion* to the madpersons, queer personae, ghosts, freaks, weirdos, imaginary friends, disembodied voices, and unReasonable others, who trespass, like stowaways or fugitives, in Reasonable modernity" (2021, 10).[8] The radical compassion that Grande, Díaz, Zamora, and Cornejo inspire is not merely a gesture of care toward their own parents, but the forging of an ethic of radical migrant mental health—one that both destigmatizes the effects of trauma and critiques the conditions that produce it. The texts examined here thus illuminate the need for immigration policy that accounts for the traumas that both compel and accompany migration.

Reyna Grande: American Dreams and Nightmares

In her second memoir, *A Dream Called Home* (2019), Grande recounts a conversation with her younger sister, Betty. A college student working to escape poverty and abuse, Reyna has traveled to her hometown of Iguala de la Independencia, Guerrero, Mexico, to convince fifteen-year-old Betty to return to the United States and stay in school. As Betty expresses her desperation to leave their mother's home, Reyna says how sorry she is: "And I meant I was sorry about everything, how immigration and separation had taken a toll on all of us, how even though our parents had emigrated from this very city to go to the U.S. to build us a house, they ended up destroying our home" (55). With this thought unspoken between the sisters, Betty asks: "Do you think things would have been different if they had never left? Do you think we would all be together as a family?" (55).

Betty's question—*did our parents do the right thing?*—haunts all of Grande's published work, fiction as well as nonfiction, which explores themes of migration and loss. Grande was two years old when her father left Iguala for the United States and four when her mother followed, leaving her and her older siblings (Mago and Carlos) with their paternal grandmother, who neglected and abused them. When Grande was nine, her father returned for Grande's older siblings, and Mago convinced him to take Grande as well, even though he correctly believed her too young to make the journey. (Because of Grande's difficulty keeping up, the family was caught and turned back twice, finally crossing on their third attempt, with Grande carried much of the way on her father's back.) While reuniting with her father improved Grande's life in many ways—food security, education, medical care—it did not end the abuse, which her father (who also experienced abuse as a child) continued. These biographical facts help to contextualize the ambivalent grappling with the aftermath of migration that characterizes Grande's writing.

One explanation for the mainstream success of Grande's work, especially her memoirs, lies in the way her life story—brought to the United States as a child, first in her family to graduate from college, now a successful writer—seems to align with an American Dream narrative. After publishing two novels, *Across a Hundred Mountains* (2006) and *Dancing with Butterflies* (2009), Grande wrote the story of her childhood in Mexico, journey to the United States, and subsequent life in the United States in two memoirs, *The Distance between Us* (2012) and *A Dream Called Home*. These latter two books, in particular, received both critical acclaim and commercial success, and *The Distance between Us* was reissued in an edition for young readers (2016). Indeed, Grande's publisher (Simon and Schuster) often presents her work as an American Dream story; the company website bills *A Dream Called Home* as the "inspiring account of one woman's quest to find her place in America as a first-generation Latina university student and aspiring writer determined to build a new life for her family one fearless word at a time" (Simon and Schuster, n.d.). Yet Grande's ambivalent representation of her parents sits uneasily with this marketing strategy, undermining what Alvarado calls the "recourse to assimilationist appeals for respectability"

(2018, 3) that American Dream narratives reinforce. For this reason, I read Grande's memoirs as a complex negotiation with the American Dream, registering the American Dream as a threat to migrant health and wellbeing even as they also reproduce it.

In an interview with Patricia M. García, Grande asserts two goals for her writing. First: "I want to inspire compassion and understanding towards immigrants . . . I feel that many times people are anti-immigrant because of ignorance, because they honestly don't know, because they haven't been exposed to the issue from a perspective that highlights the human cost and heartbreak" (García 2017, 195). Second: "I wanted to offer immigrant youth . . . a mirror in which they could see themselves" (197). Although both goals are politically urgent given the virulent anti-immigrant hostility of our cultural moment, it is worth asking how compatible they actually are. Consider, for instance, two passages from *The Distance between Us*. The first concerns a violent confrontation between her parents; a bystander intervenes and is accidentally shot with her father's gun: "Luckily for my father, the man did not die. Luckily for my father, he was allowed voluntary deportation, instead of getting thrown in prison. Within a week, he had managed to sneak across the border and resumed his life in the United States as if nothing had ever happened" (2012, 86). The second describes her mother: "Even though we had suggested that she learn English and find herself a better job, my mother insisted on living the way she had lived in Mexico or the way she had lived when she was still undocumented. She refused to learn English and how to drive a car. She refused to look for a job that could offer her benefits—such as medical insurance and a pension plan, and where she could finally get off welfare" (274). The first time I taught Grande's memoir, I was nervous about how it would be received; I have myself experienced intense emotional distress (as someone who grew up on public assistance) when students have made callous comments in class about lazy people living on welfare at US taxpayers' expense, and I worried about whether Grande's unflinching portrayal of her own parents could inspire conversations in class that would be harmful to students with life experiences similar to those she depicts.[9] I mention these concerns not as a critique of Grande, but rather to suggest that even as Grande purports to imagine two kinds of readers for her work—the outsider to the immigrant experience and the immigrant youth—she ultimately privileges the second, prioritizing immigrant readers' need for complex stories about their lives even if they don't conform to the demands of respectability politics.

To explain the importance of this move, I'd like to highlight another passage from *The Distance between Us*, in which Reyna reads Sandra Cisneros's novel *The House on Mango Street* for the first time and is riveted by a chapter about a young woman with an abusive father: "When I got to the chapter titled 'Sally,' I broke down. I shook with an intense sadness and helplessness, and tears burned my eyes. . . . I reread the chapter and with every word I felt that Cisneros was reaching out and talking to me. I felt a connection to this author, this person, whom I had never met" (2012, 306). What Grande describes in this passage is what Alvarado calls "a shared sense of being . . . in negative relation to majoritarian publics" (2018, 6), a sense of affinity for Cisneros's character that emerges not from an inspirational story of overcoming but from shared fear and desire for escape. Grande never re-solves her ambivalence toward her parents. Instead, she ends *The Distance between Us* with a scene at her father's deathbed, in which she confronts two versions of her father—"the violent, alcoholic one" (321) and "the one who taught me to dream big" (321)—and concludes: "*You made me who I am*" (322; original italics). Claudia A. Anguiano and Karma R. Chávez note that US immigration discourse is so conservative that "undocumented youth have limited resources available in the construction of their narratives" (2011, 83) and often tell stories implicitly affirming "that only immigrants with desirable characteristics such that they possess have earned the right to formally belong in the United States" (97). By refusing to edit out details about her parents that don't align with such rhetoric, Grande might sacrifice some of the "anti-immigration" readers she claims to court but prioritizes readers in need of a story that doesn't make belonging in the United States contingent on "desirable characteristics." As Cisneros did for Grande with the character of Sally, Grande offers the representation of her parents as a means of expanding what Anguiano and Chávez might call the "narrative resources" available to youth in similar circumstances.

Grande pairs critique of her parents with a structural critique of the geopolitical circumstances they navigate. As she tells García: "I have no qualms about criticizing Mexico and the Mexican government for its cor-ruption, impunity, and violation of human rights. I also did not hesitate to criticize the U.S. government's role in the violence and poverty that is raging across my native country" (García 2017, 188–89). Here it is useful to contrast Grande with the aforementioned Nazario, who—as Puga and Espinosa (2020, 273) point out—urges migrant mothers not to leave their children while failing to address the "global economic and cultural forces that demand cheap labor and vulnerable bodies." Both of Grande's memoirs mention the political context of migration, from the 1982 Mexican peso crisis, to the 2014 kidnapping of forty-three students at the Ayotzinapa Rural Teachers' College in Iguala, to the repeated failures of the US government to enact the DREAM Act. They also depict in vivid detail the dangers that poverty poses to those who experience it; Grande describes vulnerability to dangerous accidents and health crises (including the scars on her sister's face from a game of hide-and-seek gone awry, the scars on her mother's hands from a workplace accident, her cousin Catalina's death by drowning, and her own experiences with scorpion bites and roundworms). Although US border enforcement has made crossing the border an undeniably dangerous endeavor, it is also clear that staying in Mexico was neither economically viable nor safe for Grande's family. In the epilogue to *The Distance between Us*, Grande writes about working as a teacher in the Los Angeles Unified School District and recognizing the effects of family separation in her students: "The cycle of leaving children behind has not ended. Nor will it end, as long as there is poverty" (2012, 320). The reason parents migrate, she makes clear, is not lack of judgment but lack of alternatives.

In this regard, the prologue to *The Distance between Us*, which invokes the Mexican folktale of La Llorona, is particularly significant: "My father's mother, Abuela Evila, liked to scare us with stories of La Llorona, the weeping woman who roams the canal and steals children away. She would say that if we didn't behave, La Llorona would take us far away where we would never see our parents again" (2012, 3). By invoking La Llorona—who infamously sacrificed her own children and is eternally punished for it—Grande might seem to be setting up a story of children abandoned or endangered by their parents. Yet, as Domino Renee Perez reminds us, La Llorona herself is "an avatar of social and cultural conflict" (2008, 13), one frequently repurposed by Mexican American writers for heterogeneous political ends. Grande, it turns out, uses La Llorona to introduce her story's true villain: "Neither of my grandmothers told us that there is something more powerful than La Llorona—a power that takes away parents, not children. It is called The United States" (2012, 3). By beginning her first memoir in this way, Grande imbues the United States—and its American Dream—with the qualities of a traditional La Llorona story: grief, loss, betrayal. And although she ultimately ends the memoir by answering in the affirmative a question she asks repeatedly—"If I had known what life with my father would be like, would I have still followed him to El Otro Lado?" (322)—La Llorona's signature themes nonetheless haunt the story Grande tells of her life in the United States.

In this way, Grande attempts to strike a difficult balance between affirming her parents' decision to migrate and not reifying myths of the United States as a land of opportunity. Whereas Nazario has been rightfully critiqued for her "contention that Latin American mothers should remain in their home countries, no matter how dire their economic circumstances" (Puga and Espinosa 2020, 245), Alicia Muñoz and Ariana E. Vigil note that Grande also takes a risk by portraying her younger self as invested in upward mobility through education and work: "For readers critical of US immigration policy and the social and racial stratification it causes, this 'buying into' the American Dream on the part of Grande can be perplexing" (2019, 233). It is important, then, to note that not only does Grande depict her life in the United States as marked by success and opportunity, she also depicts it as marked by harrowing scenes of domestic abuse: "The home that she inhabits in the US is ruled by fear—of [her father's] abuse and of their undocumented status" (A. Muñoz and Vigil 2019, 220). In her first memoir, Grande aligns the representation of her father with her life in the United States, and thus with economic advancement and social mobility, but the detailed descriptions of her father's abuse also mean that her perception of the American Dream is inevitably infused with violence: "When my father beat me, and in his drunken stupor called me a pendeja and an hija de la chingada, I held on to the vision of the future he had given me during his sober moments. I thought about that vision when the blows came, because the father who beat me . . . wasn't the same father who told me that one day I would be somebody in this country" (2012, 250–51). While this passage appears to differentiate the abusive father from the one who instills the American Dream, the rest of the book makes starkly clear that these two fathers are indeed the very same person.

In her second memoir, *A Dream Called Home*, Grande redirects this representation of the American Dream; here, it becomes a weapon she wields to enact revenge on her parents. Two scenes in particular illustrate this point. The first takes place at Reyna's college graduation. She has won an essay competition to honor her beloved teacher from Pasadena City College, Diana Savas, and is invited to read the essay at commencement: "As I spoke about my father's alcoholism, the abuse I had experienced at home, and the lack of support, what mattered most to me was honoring Diana. . . . I did not consider how it would affect my father, who despite his broken English, knew perfectly well what I was saying about him to the hundreds of strangers at the ceremony" (2019, 135–36). Afterward, Reyna notes "the pain so openly displayed on his face, a vulnerability I rarely got to see" (136–37) and wants to apologize, but she finds herself unable to; instead, she relates that her father, despite his hurt and shame, shakes her teacher's hand and thanks her. Another scene recounts how Reyna's mother begins visiting her after she purchases her first home in South Central Los Angeles, befriends a neighborhood fruit vendor, and starts her own business selling used clothing, furniture, and household goods from Reyna's front yard, causing Reyna to fret about the "curb appeal" (293) of her home. When her mother finds Reyna's compost bin and mistakes it for trash, Reyna can no longer contain her irritation and forces her mother to go back into the trash to retrieve her kitchen scraps. It is Reyna's younger sister who informs her of how this affects their mother: "Later that night when I spoke with Betty, the first thing she told me was that my mother had called her and told her I made her dig through the trash. 'She was crying,' Betty said" (299). Yet again, even as Reyna acknowledges to Betty that she has done "a shitty thing" (299), she does not apologize to her mother.

Although Grande unflinchingly depicts her parents' abuse and neglect, she also details the abuse and neglect they experienced as children, and for this reason these scenes in *A Dream Called Home* of Reyna shaming her parents are difficult to read; her choice to emphasize her own refusal on both occasions to apologize heightens this difficulty. Grande does not depict these moments as the moral equivalent of her parents' actions (they certainly cannot be described as *abuse* in the same way as her descriptions of her father punching her in the face), but they are clearly marked in the text as moments of self-critique. Furthermore, it is significant that these moments align with American Dream milestones: college graduation and the purchase of a home. Conservative rhetoric on immigration often indicates that the economic advantages of migration are "not worth it" because they entail family dissolution, thus presenting what Puga and Espinosa call "a false binary—family unity versus material security—and a false hierarchy— love trumps money—that recycles simplistic fantasies of poor-but-happy fictional families" (2020, 243). In these passages, Grande shifts this rhetoric: it is not her parents' act of migration but her own internalization of the American Dream that separates parents and children.

Grande's representation of her parents neither disavows them nor ignores their harmful actions. Instead, they exemplify Bruce's radical compassion, which "persists even and especially toward beings who are the objects of contempt and condemnation from dominant value systems" (2020, 10). To conclude, I note that one of the mechanisms that makes possible this radical compassion is the Immigration Reform and Control Act (IRCA) of

1986, which took effect the year after Grande arrived in the United States and enabled her family to formalize their immigration status and eventually become US citizens. For this reason, Grande is able to travel across the US-Mexico border and to remain in close contact with relatives in Mexico, a fact that she highlights in both of her memoirs. This gives Grande access to her family history, which in turn has a significant impact on the shape of her narrative. For instance, in *A Dream Called Home*, Grande recounts the last time she saw her paternal grandmother alive, on the same trip to Iguala where Betty asks Reyna whether their parents should have stayed. The grandmother, who is experiencing dementia, begins pinching her arms and claiming to be eaten by maggots, and Reyna's aunt explains that when the grandmother was a child and infected with measles, she had to pull maggots out of her own open sores because her parents had no access to medical treatment. As Reyna says goodbye for the last time to the grand-mother who first abused her father and then abused her, she decides "to think instead about that little girl who had to pull maggots out of her own flesh and, despite all odds, had found the will to live" (2019, 65). Because Grande places this story early in the memoir, the subsequent descriptions of her difficulties with her parents are always told to the reader in light of this story about the intergenerational trauma of extreme poverty. Yet while the IRCA makes it possible for Grande to return to Mexico and revisit this history, those who have migrated to the United States since 1986 do not have this option. As Marion Christina Rohrleitner notes, the IRCA is often remembered as an amnesty program for undocumented immigrants, but it also "initiated the militarisation of the U.S.-Mexico border" (2017, 42) in ways that have profoundly changed both the experience of those migrating afterward and the representation of migration in Latinx literature. In the remaining sections of this chapter, I examine representations that foreclose the perspective Grande offers, including the story of Junot Díaz's character Yunior, whose father eventually abandons him, and the post-IRCA migration stories of Javier Zamora and Karla Cornejo Villavicencio.

Junot Díaz: Reading Hopelessly

Like Grande, Dominican writer Junot Díaz and his most famous character (Yunior) are left behind as children when their fathers migrate to the United States; both also eventually join their fathers and become writers. Yunior is the narrator of three of Díaz's published books: a novel (*The Brief Wondrous*

Life of Oscar Wao [2007]) and two short story collections (*Drown* [1996] and *This Is How You Lose Her* [2012]). Unlike in Grande's memoirs, however, Yunior's father is not a significant part of his adult life; instead, Papi (as Yunior calls him) goes from being an overbearing (abusive, oppressive, philandering) presence in Díaz's work to simply disappearing after he abandons his family. And just as the trauma arising from Papi's domestic abuse and abandonment remains unresolved in Díaz's work, also unresolved are critical debates surrounding Díaz himself that focus on whether the author and his work deconstruct or perpetuate a damaging model of masculinity.

Even before 2018, writing about Díaz's fiction required addressing these debates; in recent years, this is even more the case. In April 2018, the *New Yorker* published an essay by Díaz entitled "The Silence," in which he detailed the experience of being raped as a child and its ongoing impact; before this publication, women and queer writers of color had already been telling stories about Díaz's aggressive behavior toward them—making unwanted sexual advances, dismissing their work, and bullying them—at readings and in writing workshops, but the stories received heightened attention after "The Silence."[10] As Yomaira C. Figueroa-Vásquez notes, these accusations "add a critical dimension to how we read Díaz's work, and how we link the impact of his work and actions to the bodies and lives of women of color" (2020, 79), making it impossible to discuss Díaz's work without also discussing the controversy. Although a number of institutions with which Díaz is affiliated—including the Massachusetts Institute of Technology, the *Boston Review*, and the board of the Pulitzer Prize—investigated his actions and decided to maintain ties with him, the ethics of writing about and teaching his work remain thorny (Chasman and Cohen 2018; Flood 2018; Romo 2018). As the literary critic Maia Gil'Adí writes, in the most ambitious effort yet to grapple with the fallout from these allegations, the controversy prompts "the question of how literary scholars begin to think about the intersection of race and gender through an author who has been at the forefront of anti-sexist and anti-racist work while also seemingly performing in a manner antithetical to some of these progressive ideologies" (2020, 513).[11] The analysis I offer here—of the short stories "Fiesta 1980" and "Negocios" from Díaz's debut short story collection, *Drown* (1996)—is my attempt to grapple with the work of a writer who both theorizes trauma in his work and perpetuates it in his life. While many discussions of trauma in Díaz's work focus on sexual trauma, I address instead the trauma of family separation, arguing that Díaz offers an important entry point for thinking about the denigration of migrant parents not despite but because of the concerns raised about Díaz himself.

My current thinking about Díaz's work is informed not only by Gil'Adí's call to reassess the idea that "texts by people of color are inherently political and promote social justice" (2020, 512), but also by Therí Alyce Pickens's mad Black theory, which asks scholars of race and disability to risk examining race and disability together without prioritizing the search for liberation in the texts they read. As Pickens reminds us: "The material conditions for celebration and agency require material resources not available to everyone, and mere knowledge of one's situation cannot be proxy for freedom from it" (2019, 35). When the controversy surrounding Díaz led me to put aside his work for several years, it left a gaping hole in my syllabi as well as in my plans for this book. As I have noted elsewhere, Díaz's work richly depicts the links between racial health disparities and the racialization of disability (Minich 2016); revising this argument in light of the publication of Jasbir K. Puar's fundamental book *The Right to Maim* (2017), I would now say that Díaz's work maps the dimensions of debility without an accompanying sense of disability pride. Teaching Puar's elaboration of debility without recourse to Díaz's vivid depictions of how environmental injustice, physical labor, and poverty are lived in the body is challenging, especially because undergraduate students do (still) respond so well to Díaz's writing, and the prospect of writing about family separation without recourse to a canonical text in Latinx literature felt diminishing. My earlier writing on Díaz focuses on the character of Rafa, Yunior's older brother; I note that Rafa's death of cancer (which is linked to environmental contamination at the site of his first home in the United States) is never made redemptive, but I still give in to the desire for emancipation and social justice that Gil'Adí and Pickens regard so skeptically, holding out hope of redemption for Yunior. Now, in light of the allegations against Díaz, I ask what it might mean to read his work without that hope.

Pursuing this line of inquiry feels risky. (For this reason, my language throughout this section is more tentative and speculative than in much of this book.) First, there is the risk of wading back into Díaz criticism. My prior writing on Díaz could be characterized as part of what Gil'Adí refers to as "a form of hagiography" (2020, 509). In attempting to nuance that writing now, I risk angering friends and fellow feminist literary critics who have come to Díaz's defense as well as friends and fellow feminist literary critics who point out that perhaps Díaz has already taken up enough space in our writings and our syllabi and should be left alone (if not outright canceled). Second, there is the risk of asking why I still feel so compelled to teach and write about Díaz's work, even as I recognize his behavior as harmful. Here I find myself hailed by the questions posed by Dixa Ramírez (2018) in her response to the Díaz controversy: "I want to emphasize how many girls, Latina and otherwise, are taught that their bodies and thoughts do not belong to them. . . . How does this training shape our sense, even our sense as trained literary critics, of what literature matters? Even beyond which writers the biased literary and academic world celebrates, how does it shape what we *enjoy*?" Is the fact that I do—still—enjoy reading, teaching, and writing about Díaz an indication of my own internalized misogyny? Finally, I am about to commit a sin that literary critics are forever cautioning our first-year students against: conflating author and character. For I now see Díaz—both the Díaz of "The Silence" and the Díaz who has yet to offer an apology for his behavior that satisfies his critics and accusers—as a potential vision of what might happen to Yunior after Díaz's books end.[12] My previous writing on Díaz clings desperately to the hope that "Yunior, unlike Rafa, might find a different masculinity" (Minich 2016, 53); knowing now what I know about Díaz's behavior, I no longer have this hope. And yet, if I am invested in arguing here for Bruce's notion of radical compassion— particularly in the service of imagining a framework for enacting radical mental health—where better to go than to a character with whom I fear my own relationship is now permanently damaged?

My previous writing on Díaz has addressed the ways in which *physical* disability and illness have shaped the lives of writer and character. What I have not addressed is the fact that both Yunior and Díaz also experience trauma symptoms, to which Yunior rarely alludes directly. Indeed, Yunior's suppression of his own trauma means that a much more defining feature of Díaz's work is the trauma inflicted on women; as Tiffany Lethabo King and others have observed, much of Díaz's work does not focus directly on his own trauma but instead "transfers (and projects) his experiences of rape and sexual violation onto the bodies of Black and Indigenous women" (2019, 48). I have chosen to focus on "Fiesta 1980" and "Negocios" because these stories are unique in Díaz's body of work for situating the physical effects of trauma on *Yunior's* body ("Fiesta 1980") and for linking that trauma directly to family separation ("Negocios").

"Fiesta 1980" describes a party at the home of Yunior's Tía Yrma, who has finally made it to the United States three years after Yunior's arrival. The party is an ominous event for Yunior, due to the fact that his family must travel to it in the vw van that Papi has recently purchased: "Brand-new, lime-green, and bought to impress. Oh, we were impressed, but me, every time I was in that vw and Papi went above twenty miles an hour, I vomited. I'd never had trouble with cars before—that van was my curse" (1996, 27). The plot of the story follows the family preparing to leave, driving to the party, attending the festivities, and driving home, interspersed with Yunior's memories of how he started vomiting and the times Papi had taken him to visit the Puerto Rican woman with whom he is having an affair. In the story, Yunior also describes his father's physical abuse and his desire to be close to his father:

> I met the Puerto Rican woman right after Papi had gotten the van. He was taking me on short trips, trying to cure me of my vomiting. It wasn't really working but I looked forward to our trips, even though at the end of each one I'd be sick. These were the only times me and Papi did anything together. When we were alone he treated me much better, like maybe I was his son or something. (34–35)

Yunior's vomiting is never explained but is simply narrated alongside the facts of his everyday life, being routinely hit by his father and forced to lie to his mother about the Puerto Rican woman. In this sense, the story aligns with Angela M. Carter's (2021) understanding of trauma as an "embodied, affective structure [that] is specific, not to the horrendousness of an event or events, but rather to the debilitating sociopolitical responses and the overlapping attributes of instability that so often accompany it." Yunior's trauma cannot be explained by a single cause but arises from his father's long absence in his childhood, from the coerced intimacy of concealing his father's infidelity, from the physical and emotional violence perpetrated against him by his father and brother, and from the sexual and emotional violence perpetrated against him by other men. None of these histories are directly named by Yunior or his family in the text, even as their effects are evident and his entire family is focused on finding a remedy for his mysterious and apparently incurable vomiting.[13]

"Negocios" is Yunior's attempt to imagine his father's life during the years of their separation, when Papi arrived in the United States with the intention to overstay a tourist visa, struggled to make a living, and married another woman to secure the US citizenship that eventually enabled him to bring the family to New Jersey. Several critics, including me, have read this story as Yunior's effort to extend compassion to Papi. Moving in a slightly different direction, Caminero-Santangelo argues that the story "fills in some of the explanatory gaps about how Yunior and his family got from the Dominican Republic to the United States" (2016, 117)—specifically, how Papi's infidelity legitimated the family's migration. What is particularly compelling about Caminero-Santangelo's interpretation is her observation that Yunior "works hard to distinguish Papi's situation from that of other (Mexican and Central American) undocumented immigrants, and instead insistently groups him with 'legal' Caribbeans" (117), thus suggesting a "profound anxiety (on Yunior's part, at least) surrounding issues of legality/legitimacy vis-à-vis the patriarchal nuclear family" (119). In this sense, Yunior's effort to extend compassion to his father also entails distancing himself from others. For this reason, I have come to believe that *Drown* instantiates "the dangers of desire for normative inclusion that will require repudiation of other abjects if seeking out proper subject status" (Alvarado 2018, 9). Just as Yunior famously disavows his own sexual and gendered abjection within intimate relationships, displacing it onto the women he treats so badly, he also disavows his own intimacy with the legalized abjection of undocumented status, displacing it onto migrants whose trajectories he differentiates from that of his family.

Although it is hardly a groundbreaking critical insight to suggest that Yunior has intimacy issues, this fact has not been discussed in relation to migration and family separation. This is not to argue that family separation is "more" (or "less") traumatic than Yunior's experiences with physical/emotional abuse and sexual violence but rather to note that attending to family separation *in addition to* the other sources of trauma in Yunior's life supports a theory of trauma that attends less to the traumatizing event and more to its consequences.[14] As Deborah R. Vargas has argued, Yunior's intimate relationships—beginning with his father and extending to his lovers—are characterized by *surplus love*, or "the residue of heteronormative constructions of love as dual-partnered, monogamous, reproductive, and always aspiring to remain on normative time" (2016, 356). While Vargas's focus is not on Yunior but on his lovers, whom she refuses to treat as "mere victims of Yunior's and Rafa's sexist misogyny, or as pure radical transgressors" (2016, 357), her analysis is apt for Yunior as well, who never achieves normative domesticity and is neither purely a victim nor purely a hero. Yunior's efforts to "negotiate, reimagine, repurpose, and at times willfully fail to abide by" (Vargas 2016, 356) normative domestic arrangements certainly cannot be described solely in terms of radical transgression, with the liberatory implications contained therein, because they often involve hurting women in typically misogynist ways. Yet Yunior is not only a man who treats his lovers as surplus, he is also the recipient of his father's surplus love, a love first made surplus when his father—due to the exigencies of US immigration policies—marries and has children with another woman. Yunior thus embodies Pickens's reminder that "mere exposure of oppression is not only not emancipatory but can also be detrimental, [that] demonstration and acknowledgement of one's various intersecting socially marginalized positions does not equal political agency" (2019, 31). If Yunior's story fails to be emancipatory, it is because of the ways in which he insistently disavows his own abjection—his connection both to other migrant children who share the same disrupted relationships to their parents *and* to the lovers he treats as sexually abject.

Many critical studies of Díaz's work are affixed to the "recuperation and resistance" model that Pickens (2019, 25) critiques, recuperating Yunior as a figure who exposes the global injustices of racial capitalism and therefore offers possibilities for resistance. Elda María Román has observed something different in Yunior's story. If we read Díaz's books in chronological order, she notes, "there is a structural rise occurring over the arc of these texts; . . . together they constitute an upward mobility narrative, one of the most frequently occurring narratives in U.S. literature, and one that tends to get ignored or vilified in studies of Latina/o literature" (2017, 103).[15] Román uses this observation to interrogate how the skepticism directed at upward mobility narratives in Latinx studies leads critics to overlook the insights they offer; as a scholar of disability studies (a field that is similarly skeptical of overcoming narratives), I wonder if Román's insight might also lead us to interrogate how ignoring or vilifying the overcoming narrative can similarly preclude meaningful engagement. In the previous section, I elaborated how Grande at times replicates an American Dream story even as she also depicts that narrative as a source of migrant trauma. In the case of Díaz, I wonder if contrasting the "structural rise" of Yunior's story against his lingering trauma symptoms can prompt us to question the social mandate to overcome trauma. (In other words, is *overcoming* the only response people should have to trauma?) Furthermore, while many of Díaz's defenders have insisted on a critical distance between Díaz and Yunior, suggesting that Díaz uses Yunior to illuminate and deconstruct misogyny, I wonder whether that critical distance is really essential for feminist engagement with Díaz's work. (In other words, does Díaz *himself* have to be feminist for feminists to find reasons to read and teach his work?) Grande's books are deeply compelling because she offers a model for reckoning with trauma, but perhaps what is most powerful in Díaz's work is that he forces us to confront what happens when reckoning is withheld.

Of the many think pieces and hot takes to emerge from the Díaz controversy, one that I found particularly moving was an account by the journalist Karina Maria Cabreja (2018), who interviewed Díaz in 2016 and posed to him a series of "questions that stemmed from obsessing over every piece of literary work he'd ever published." Cabreja's account contains no salacious details or horrifying stories; instead, it is the relatively mundane story of a person approaching someone she admires and being treated dismissively: "Junot Díaz was not respectful to me. He was condescending, sarcastic, and mean; that's the truth." While many of Díaz's defenders have pointed out that he was effectively raked over the coals for behavior that white writers of his stature routinely engage in, it is also true that his behavior—especially because it has been repeatedly directed to people who are feminine, queer, and/or disabled—isn't behavior befitting someone we hold up as a champion for social justice. As with Yunior, whose story of success masks a violent disavowal of those whose sexual and legal abjection hits too close to home, many of us (me included) have been too tempted to read in Díaz's work a successful model for dismantling the trauma of profound social injustice rather than a complex accounting of how it is possible to both critique and wield power.

Reading Díaz without succumbing to this temptation may also have implications for how those of us with US citizenship continue to grapple with the ongoing harm of family separation policies enacted in our names. Thousands of children and parents have been harmed in the interest of "securing our border," and their stories will continue to unfold for decades. There will no doubt be stories of heroic overcoming, packaged to make us feel better about the abuse, and there will also be stories of traumatized people who go on to do ugly things, packaged to convince us that their suffering was inconsequential or even deserved. Reading Díaz through the lens of Bruce's radical compassion—by which I mean both reading his character Yunior *and* reading Díaz himself as a writer "with a deep and intensely articulated self-awareness about misogyny who still somehow participates in it" (Loofbourow 2018)—enables us to exercise the critical tools we will need to probe both of these stories. Bruce reminds us that radical compassion "is a mode of care—not celebration, not romanticization, not endorsement, not enjoyment" (2021, 81). Bruce helps me to think that it is possible to care for Díaz—as a person whose traumatic experiences include family separation, physical and emotional abuse, and sexual violence, and as a writer who negotiates these experiences in his work—without celebrating, romanticizing, endorsing, or enjoying the ways in which he and his work also inflict trauma. Caring for both Díaz and Yunior—as well as for Díaz's readers, critics, and accusers—means to seriously engage with his work in all its aspects: the ways in which it, as Figueroa-Vásquez beautifully puts it, "allows the reader to bear witness to the ways in which coloniality exerts power over and commits violence upon bodies deemed to be insignificant" (2020, 79), as well as the ways in which it (and he) exert that same power and commit that same violence.

To conclude this section, I'd like to emphasize the longing for his father that Yunior expresses throughout *Drown*, but especially in "Fiesta 1980" and "Negocios." In "Fiesta 1980," Yunior confesses: "Our fights didn't bother me too much. I still wanted him to love me, something that never seemed strange or contradictory until years later, when he was out of our lives" (Díaz 1996, 27). In "Negocios," Yunior ends the story by imagining his father's actions on the day he returns to the Dominican Republic to reunite with his family: "The first subway station on Bond would have taken him to the airport and I like to think that he grabbed that first train, instead of what was more likely true, that he had gone out to [his friend] Chuito's first, before flying south to get us" (208). These lines, of course, explain Yunior's surplus love, as they record his own awareness of himself as the recipient of his father's surplus love. And yet they also, in the wake of recent reassessments of Díaz's work, suggest to me something about our reading practices as cultural critics: the ways in which we, too, sometimes become as enamored with the texts we analyze as Yunior does with his father, inserting into them things we "like to think" instead of highlighting what is "more likely true."

Javier Zamora: Mad Diaspora

The family separation depicted in Javier Zamora's 2017 autobiographical poetry collection *Unaccompanied* is not the singular event of Zamora's parents' departure from El Salvador, but an ongoing process that begins before the poet's birth with the Salvadoran Civil War.[16] The separations depicted in the text thus proliferate and ricochet against one another: Javier's grandfather (a military officer) brings the war home to his wife and daughters; Javier's uncle Israel (a dissident) is disappeared after a death squad murders his fiancée; his father flees the war when Javier is two; his mother flees the war's immediate aftermath when Javier is four; Javier leaves his grandmother at age nine to join his parents; deportations continue to separate his aunts and cousins. These separations reveal US and Salvadoran national sovereignties as both destabilizing and destabilized by familial bonds; in this way, *Unaccompanied* instantiates recent arguments from María Josefina Saldaña-Portillo about US–Central American political boundaries and from Bruce about the intersections of madness and diaspora. Saldaña-Portillo argues that "Central American violence demonstrates the artificiality of bounded citizenship and its liberal promise of security within nation-state sovereignties, as refugees arriving at the US border requesting asylum make evident the contingent nature of our security on their insecurity" (2019, 1). Bruce, meanwhile, emphasizes how madness and diaspora both "transgress normative arrangements—of the sane and sovereign, in turn" (2021, 17). Whereas the previous sections focused on a myth of US cultural citizenship—the American Dream of overcoming—as a threat to migrant wellbeing, this section focuses on US citizenship itself as a maddening (both rage-inducing and psychologically damaging) political construction.

The structure of Zamora's book reflects its subject: composed of six sections, all unnumbered and untitled, that move backward and forward in time, *Unaccompanied* suggests a permeability between Zamora's present and his family's past, as well as between Central America and the United States. The first and last sections consist of only one poem each: "To Abuelita Neli," which opens the book, addresses the grandmother who raised Zamora and to whom he cannot return due to his undocumented status in the United States; "June 10, 1999," which ends the collection and is named for the day of Zamora's arrival in the United States, juxtaposes his current travels as a poet with memories of his migration. In between these poems are four sections, consisting of nine to twelve poems each, that respectively examine his physical and emotional movement between La Herradura, El Salvador, and San Rafael, California; his family's experience of the war; his early childhood in El Salvador; and his arrival in the United States.

In interviews, Zamora stresses the relationship between the form of his poems and the circumstances that produce them. He tells the *New Yorker*, for instance, that the fragmented quality of a poem offers him a way to reconstruct events that occurred before his birth or that he cannot reliably recall, like the six weeks of his journey after crossing Guatemala: "The memories got more sparse at that point. . . . From Guatemala on, everything turned into poems" (Blitzer 2017).[17] In a conversation with the poet-scholar Deborah Paredez, Zamora juxtaposes the brevity of a poem against the uncontainable experience of trauma, loss, and uncertainty: "The literal shortness of poetry, its ability to fit on one page, that 'completeness' of a first draft, spoke to me. . . . For me, a teenager suffering through the complexities of being undocumented, this ability to finish something and ponder it and later re-vise it and revise it until I was happy with it, gave me a control I could not enjoy in my day-to-day life" (Paredez 2017). Both statements capture how the precarity of life in El Salvador, the migrant journey, and undocumented existence in the United States expose what Saldaña-Portillo calls "the arti-ficiality of the promise of universal, democratic citizenship" (2019, 10). In effect, the individual poems of *Unaccompanied* offer the illusion of a sin-gular event that coalesces into a defined narrative, but the way the poems come together reveals a much more disjointed set of partially remembered/partially reconstructed episodes, thus exposing the instability—political, economic, personal, and psychological—produced by US interventions in El Salvador.

The "historic and ontological role that Central American citizens' insecurity has played in securing our security as US citizens" (Saldaña-Portillo 2019, 2) is evident in the evocation of US presidents throughout the collection. The first appears in the opening poem, "To Abuelita Neli," which expresses the grief of being unable to visit his grandmother in El Salvador: "Today, this country/chose its first black president. Maybe he changes things" (Zamora 2017, 3). Because the collection was published in 2017—after Obama was dubbed the Deporter-in-Chief by immigration activists (Epstein 2014), after his failure to enact permanent policies to pro-tect migrants, after the election of a successor who sought to obliterate even the symbolic achievements of Obama's tenure in office—this line evokes not hope but disappointment, a reminder of what has *not* changed. The poem "To President-Elect," from the second section, appears to address Donald Trump, but the titular president-elect is not named, reminding the reader that presidents of both major US political parties have overseen disastrous migration policies. This poem taunts the president-elect with the permeability of the southern border: "there's a hole in the wall, yes,/you think right now ¿no one's running?" (2017, 15). The final line describes the speaker and his fellow migrants being picked up by a coyote network in southern Arizona, who greet the migrants by saying "*sobreviviste carnal*," to which the speaker replies: "Yes, we over-lived" (15). Here a conjoining of English words ("over-live") offers a too-literal translation for the Spanish word *sobrevivir* ("to survive"). Migrant life is thus depicted not as inspi-rational resilience but as excess, calling to mind what Bruce designates as the "mad diaspora" of racial capitalism: "a scattering of captives across sovereign borders and over bodies of water; an upheaval and dispersal of persons flung far from home; and an emergence of unprecedented diasporic subjectivities, ontologies, and possibilities that transgress national and rational norms" (2021, 2–3). Finally, the poem "Disappeared" consists only of a list of those responsible for violence in El Salvador, including Salvadoran and US politicians and institutions, and including the names of George H. W. Bush, Ronald Reagan, and Jimmy Carter. While the reference to Barack Obama is contained within a poem addressed to Abuelita Neli, "To President-Elect" and "Disappeared" are positioned alongside poems focusing on familial relationships. Thus, whether directly within the poem or through its positioning alongside other poems, each of these references to US presidents functions to disrupt familial relations, highlighting how migration and family separation result not from individual choices but from geopolitical relationships between Central America and the United States.

Many poems in *Unaccompanied* trace the impact of political institutions on intimate relationships. For instance, the poems about Javier's grandfather (who is named formally, as *Don Chepe*, rather than with an affectionate name like Abuelita Neli, and who is one of the few relatives mentioned in the poems but not in the book's acknowledgments) detail how the combat training he receives via US military aid affects his family, who are forced to endure the trauma he brings home. The poem "Nocturne" makes explicit the connections among the violence of US intervention in El Salvador, domestic violence, and migration, revealing that Don Chepe "chased us/ to this country that trained him to stay quiet/when 'his boss' put prisoners in black bags,/then pushed them from the truck" (70); Zamora ends the poem by concluding that his mother, his aunts, and he are "all running/ from the sun on his machete./The moon on his gun" (71). Contradicting migration rhetorics that attempt to draw a neat line between domestic and political violence, this poem reveals their interconnections. Meanwhile, poems that depict the speaker's present-day romantic life demonstrate the way his undocumented status in the United States affects his intimate relationships. The poem "Vows," a love poem, begins by describing the "brown girl [who] wanted fifteen thousand from me/to marry her" (69), a memory "that hurt me so much to never buy rings" (69); it goes on to describe the speaker's pain at being permanently separated from his grandmother and childhood home before concluding with the speaker's desire to lie next to his lover each morning and to "dive headfirst to know/what it's like to swim in the middle of love" (69). This is a poem, then, about a speaker who loves in spite of political obstacles, but it is also about how love is indelibly and inevitably marked by geopolitical structures much larger than two intimates. These poems reveal how state intervention—whether through US military aid to El Salvador or through immigration policies that regulate intimate relationships—is lived and felt in the most private of domains.

A poem that coalesces these concerns is "Cassette Tape," which appears in the second section (describing the crossing). This poem consists of five stanzas: an "A" side with an opening stanza and then two more stanzas preceded by >> and << symbols to designate fast-forwarding and rewinding, and a "B" side with an opening stanza followed by another >> (fast-forward) stanza. The "A" side describes Zamora's journey across Mexico, being cheated by coyotes, longing both for his parents and for El Salvador. The "B" side delves into the motivations for migration. Beginning with the axiom "*You don't need more than food,/a roof, and clothes on your back*" (14), it deconstructs this, explaining emotional needs and the need to be free of violence: "I'll add Mom's warmth, the need for war to stop" (14). The >> (fast-forward) section in the "B" side depicts a scene between the speaker and his mother, in which she plays for him a song she plays for the child she babysits to help with speech development, only to begin crying: "*mijo,/sorry for leaving. I wish I could've taken you to music classes*" (14). The poem ends with his response: "*you can sing to me now*" (14). This poem mirrors both the structure of a cassette tape—with songs that narrate larger political themes interspersed with more intimate songs about interpersonal relationships—and the way family relationships themselves—marked by separation and then the immediate intimacy of reunification—can feel fast-forwarded and rewound. The final stanza, in which the speaker and his mother attempt to rebuild their relationship in the aftermath of separation, demonstrates poignantly the everyday moments of tenderness sacrificed during separation and the psychic pain for both parent and child that ensues from that sacrifice.

Unaccompanied also takes a skeptical look at the social and medical institutions in the United States tasked with the treatment of trauma. Where they are depicted in the collection, health professionals are either ineffective or harmful. For instance, in "*from* The Book I Made with a Counselor My First Week of School," the counselor's annotations on Javier's drawings reveal her inability to comprehend his experience: "Next to what might be yucca plants or a dried creek:/*Javier saw a dead coyote animal, which stank and had flies over it.* . . . I just smiled, didn't tell her, *no animal, I knew that man*" (8). Meanwhile, "Doctor's Office Visit First Week in This Country" depicts the experience of being sexually assaulted during a medical exam, an experience that—because his parents take him to the doctor—affects his relationship with his parents. The critiques of school counselors and health care workers in these poems are not simply a rejection of medicine or therapy, but an insistence on their insufficiency (at best) or active harm (at worst) in a sociopolitical context in which migration experiences are systemically misunderstood and migrant lives systemically devalued. Like disability theorist Eunjung Kim, who understands medical intervention as "a transaction and negotiation that involves various effects, including the uncertainty of gains and the possibility of harm" (2017, 10), these poems stage medical and social interventions in the United States as forms of "curative violence" (10) rather than as sources of healing. In this way, they present a much more direct critique of American Dream narratives than either Grande or Díaz, showing how harms perpetuated because of US imperial dominance continue after migration.

Named for the date of Javier's arrival in the United States, the poem "June 10, 1999," which ends the collection, stunningly condenses the themes of the book and juxtaposes the events of the speaker's journey, his life in the United States, and his grandmother's life in El Salvador. Bruce proposes a side-by-side analysis of "diasporas of blackness and madness" (2021, 183), noting that black diaspora refers not only to the aftermath of transatlantic slavery but also to that of "persecution, war, sanctuary-seeking, fugitivity, exile, carceral relocations, itinerant labor, and wanderlust" (183) while mad diaspora addresses "the scattering of mad persons from their homes by vicissitudes of foolish ships, persecution, war, institutionalization, deinstitutionalization, exile, fugitivity, dissociative fugue, carceral relocations, abandonment, and snaps and clicks, among myriad other sociopolitical and existential conditions" (183–84). Similarly, Zamora in this poem aligns the diasporic movement of Central Americans in response to US intervention in the region with "the scattering of mad persons." The poem is thirteen pages long, subdivided into twelve smaller poems that are each designated with the Roman numeral "I," so that even as the narrative of the poem moves forward as the reader turns the pages of the book, the events that comprise its plot do not move forward in linear time but instead leap forward and backward like the experience of a flashback. In this way, the poem both replicates a classic symptom of post-traumatic stress disorder and challenges an individual or medicalized notion of trauma, aligning with Ann Cvetkovich's sense that "even if the PTSD diagnosis has certain strategic merits, it is wise to remain vigilant about the hazards of converting a social problem into a medical one" (2003, 45). Although the speaker of the poem is clearly traumatized, it is also clear that his trauma—war, crossing a militarized border, and family separation—is politically constructed, so that individual healing and therapy can never be enough. At the same time, the structure of the poem also registers a deep cynicism about the possibility of political change. Recalling that the opening poem, "To Abuelita Neli," questions whether the election of Obama will change anything, it is noteworthy that the final poem (and thus the book) ends with the speaker's statement that "nothing has changed" (91). Indeed, what change there is has been negative; the poem's fourth segment reveals that Javier's parents—who came to the United States before Operation Gatekeeper militarized the border and forced migrants into dangerous desert crossings—didn't anticipate how much more difficult his crossing would be, and ends with him telling his parents: "you couldn't have known this could happen . . . no es su culpa" (82). In this way, the poem both directly addresses the discourses blaming migrant parents for the harms their children experience and also elaborates the responsibility of the US government for those harms.

Where Grande and Díaz respond to the scapegoating of migrant parents through a reassessment of the American Dream and its overcoming discourse, Zamora's poetry shows that the blame placed on migrant parents deflects the rightful recipient of blame: US foreign policy and the rights and privileges of US citizenship. Grande and Díaz certainly critique the barriers to accessing US citizenship and showcase the costs of securing it, but ultimately the narrative structure of their texts follows what is called in contemporary political discourse a recognizable "path to citizenship." Zamora, by contrast, inherits a migration story in which access to citizenship is denied at every turn. Indeed, the declaration in his opening poem that "there's no path to papers" (3) becomes an organizing principle for the book itself: individual poems describe bounded events but do not add up to a clear narrative; the collection overall refuses a coherent path toward national belonging (in either the United States or El Salvador) and instead continually returns to the migration route. The final line of the collection— "nothing has changed" (91)—thus refers not only to the poet's individual political status but to the ongoing geopolitical relationship between the United States and Central America.

Karla Cornejo Villavicencio: Mad as in Crazy/Mad as in Pissed Off

Karla Cornejo Villavicencio's *The Undocumented Americans* (2020) is the most recent of the texts discussed here and is also the most direct in its analysis of migrant health. The book interweaves the stories of undocumented people across the United States with Cornejo's own: she was born in Ecuador, left by her parents with relatives as a toddler, and flew to New York City five years later to reunite with them, ultimately graduating from Harvard and becoming a writer. All of the stories that Cornejo tells in *The Undocumented Americans* touch on migrant health in some way: the workplace health concerns of Staten Island day laborers; the 9/11 second responders who cleaned up Ground Zero and now live with cancer, lung disease, and PTSD; the lack of health insurance options for people who are undocumented; the effects of the water crisis on undocumented residents of Flint, Michigan; the trauma experienced by children whose parents are deported; and the effects of aging after a life of physical labor. Throughout, Cornejo discusses her own mental health, which she insistently links not only to her own experience of family separation but also to the conditions of precarity in which undocumented people live in the United States. In this way, she gives voice to the rage of those "subjected to heinous violence and degradation, but rarely granted recourse" (Bruce 2021, 7). Addressing the relationship between Black madness and Black rage, Bruce notes that "when black people get mad (as in *angry*), antiblack logics tend to presume they've gone mad (as in *crazy*)" (8). Cornejo, writing explicitly about both her fury at anti-immigrant policy and her mental health diagnoses, similarly seizes on this conflation of meaning and situates her book at the intersection of these two meanings of *mad*. For Cornejo, in other words, rage is a crucial mechanism for theorizing radical migrant mental health.

From the opening pages of the book, Cornejo is explicit about the impossible representational conundrum she must negotiate. On one hand, it is her status as both exceptionally accomplished and undocumented that initially gave her access to a public platform; on another, she shares the critique of Alvarado (and others) of the way calls for immigration reform often evoke "the revered, respectable, and protected figure of the student . . . despite its lack of applicability across the undocumented community and its limited implications for a diverse group identifiable under the umbrella of Latinidad" (Alvarado 2018, 3). Cornejo asserts in her introduction that DREAMers "are commendable young people, and I truly owe them my life, but they occupy outsize attention in our politics" (2020, xvi). Her goal, she continues, is to "step away from the buzzwords in immigration, the talking heads, the kids in graduation caps and gowns" (xvi–xvii) and to represent immigrants as everyday people: "Not heroes. Randoms. People. Characters" (xvii). The origins of the book lie in an anonymous article she wrote pre-DACA for the *Daily Beast* when she was about to graduate from

Harvard with no viable career options, an article that garnered the attention of agents who began begging her for a memoir: "I was angry. A *memoir?* I was twenty-one. I wasn't fucking Barbra Streisand. . . . I didn't want my first book to be a rueful tale about being a sickly Victorian orphan with tuberculosis who didn't have a social security number, which is what the agents all wanted" (xiv). She has highlighted this representational challenge in interviews as well, telling Lucas Iberico Lozada:

> DREAMer memoirs have their purpose. But that's not what I set out to write. My book is a serious work of literature. When I've done interviews, people don't ask me about literary things, people don't ask me about formal things, people don't often ask me about my influences or whether I have any training in writing or who I studied under or things like that. People just ask me about my parents leaving me in Ecuador, or what I do for self-care, things like that. It's very clear that I'm being seen through a sociological lens. (Iberico Lozada 2020)

Rather than describing Cornejo's book as a memoir, I classify it here as a chronicle, a genre theorized by the literary critic Monica Hanna with roots in US-based traditions of literary journalism and the Latin American *crónica*.[18] According to Hanna, the chronicle's journalistic aspects enable Latinx authors "to engage with and document the present, entering political discourse while entering their subjects into the historical record" (2016, 362) even as its subjective aspects reject "the notion of journalism (and historical interventions) as objective, instead highlighting subjectivity, selection, and interpretation" (362). Understanding Cornejo's work through the collective lens of the chronicle thus emphasizes her politicized approach to migrant madness.

To understand how Cornejo grapples with the conflation of mental illness and rage requires examining her insistent use of the word *crazy* throughout the text. While casual uses of the term have been critiqued for their stigmatizing effects, Cornejo has defended her use of it, stating in one interview: "The way I define crazy is not just 'mentally ill.' It's a radical term, the way that people with disabilities have used the word 'crip'" (Iberico Lozano 2020). The word first appears in the book's introduction and is from the beginning intertwined with anger:

> By this point, I had been pursuing a PhD at Yale because I needed the health insurance and had read lots of books about migrants and I hated a good number of the texts. I couldn't see my family in them,

because I saw my parents as more than laborers, more than sufferers or dreamers. I thought I could write something better, something that rang true. And I thought that I was the best person to do it. I was just crazy enough. Because if you're going to write a book about undocumented immigrants in America, the story, the full story, you have to be a little bit crazy. And you certainly can't be enamored by America, not still. That disqualifies you. (Cornejo 2020, xv)

At this point, a reader might assume that she means *crazy* in the colloquial sense: someone with an unusual perspective, perhaps, or someone prone to risk-taking. Yet even here, before Cornejo has identified herself as someone living with diagnoses of mental illness, the association between madness and rage is clear: Cornejo is angry about literature that reduces immigrants to suffering workers; this anger qualifies her to tell an untold story.

It is not until the third chapter of the book that Cornejo describes in detail the mental illnesses that establish her claim to the word *crazy*, and when she finally does so, she precedes the disclosure with a gorgeous description of her mother, who "is in the middle of a feminist awakening" (57), has become "a whole new woman, emancipated and bold" (58), and is "kind to you if you're 1) my partner or 2) a formerly abused dog" (59). Here Cornejo appears to deliberately anticipate a reader who will link her mental illness to the fact that her parents left her in Ecuador and routes this reader through a loving portrait of her mother to arrive at a discussion of mental illness:

I've always been super casual when people ask me about my parents having left me in Ecuador. . . . I don't feel anything about being left on the day-to-day but I am told by mental health experts that it has affected me. And I fought that conclusion. I denied it. I wanted to be a genius. I wanted my mental illnesses to be purely biological. I wanted to have been born wild and crazy and weird and brilliant, writing math equations in chalk on a window. Instead, therapist after therapist told me I had attachment issues related to my childhood. I left those therapists. Ghosted them. (59)

What is at stake in Cornejo's rejection of her therapists is not just her desire to be "weird and brilliant" (although by the time a reader reaches this passage, she has certainly demonstrated that she is both). What is also at stake is her *mother's* right to be "emancipated and bold"—that is, to be seen (by the reader and by therapists) as a complicated, interesting, and charming person who deserves her daughter's love and the respect of her daughter's readers, rather than simply as a victim of circumstance and poverty who was forced to abandon her daughter.

By using the past tense to relate that she "fought" her therapists' conclusions and ghosted them, Cornejo does implicitly give credence to their theory that she developed attachment issues in early childhood. However, she also underscores the role of the border enforcement policies that make life for undocumented people in the United States unnecessarily difficult: "But it's not just those early years without my parents that branded me. It's the life I've led in America as a migrant, watching my parents pursue their dream in this country and then having to deal with its carcass, witnessing the crimes against migrants carried out by the U.S. government with my hands bound. As an undocumented person, I felt like a hologram. Nothing felt secure" (59–60). In fact, while Cornejo devotes a single paragraph to the perspective of mental health professionals who note the impact of parental separation on her mental health, she devotes two full pages to the impact of the precarity she has experienced as a result of US immigration law. The treatment of migrants by the US government, she says, has made her feel crazy:

> When I was growing up, and throughout the Obama administration, . . . I felt crazy for thinking we were under attack, watching my neighbors disappear and then going to school and watching the nightly news and watching award shows and seeing no mention. I felt crazy watching the white supremacist state slowly kill my father and break my family apart. I would frantically tell everyone that there was no such thing as the American Dream but then some all-star immigrants around me who had done things "the right way" preached a different story and Americans ate that up. It all made me feel crazy. I also am crazy. Pero why? (60–61)

It is here—in the discussion of the impact of US border enforcement on migrant health—that the two meanings of *mad* at play in the text collide. "It all made me feel crazy" denotes the experience of rage that Bruce describes, of those subjected to violence without recourse to justice, whereas the next sentence—"I also am crazy"—describes the fact of having received a diagnosis of mental illness.

Ultimately, Cornejo comes to reject the stigma of mental illness, portraying herself and others who have experienced parental separation as part of an "army of mutants":

Researchers have shown that the flooding of stress hormones resulting from a traumatic separation from your parents at a young age kills off so many dendrites and neurons in the brain that it results in permanent psychological and physical changes. One psychiatrist I went to told me that my brain looked like a tree without branches.

So I just think about all the children who have been separated from their parents, and there's a lot of us, past and present, and some under more traumatic circumstances than others—like those who are in internment camps right now—and I just imagine us as an army of mutants. We've all been touched by this monster, and our brains are forever changed, and we all have trees without branches in there, and what will happen to us? Who will we become? (59–61)

Although it might be tempting to read this passage as an instantiation of "mad pride," I argue that it resonates more closely with the work of scholars like Alvarado and Jasbir K. Puar who interrogate the political uses to which pride is often put. For Alvarado, an insistence on pride can "reinforce hegemonic norms by underscoring their desirability" (2018, 10), whereas for Puar disability pride in particular can efface "the biopolitical production of precarity and (un)livability" (2017, xxiv). Even as Cornejo sardonically undermines the pathologizing language of the psychiatrist who compares her brain to a "tree without branches," she also characterizes the sociopolitical conditions that have shaped her brain as the touch of a "monster." In the passages that describe Cornejo's experience of mental illness (and particularly those that describe feeling crazy), *The Undocumented Americans* advances what I have been calling throughout this book an ethic of radical health: an insistence on destigmatizing pathologized bodies and minds without celebrating the injustices that produce them.

It is important to note, however, that this theoretical work has come at an emotional cost for Cornejo herself. In an essay published in *The Nation* just as I finished the first draft of this chapter, an essay that reflected on her life in the eighteen months since the publication of *The Undocumented Americans*, Cornejo (2021) writes of her own exhaustion with the topic it covers: "I have a dream, a total fantasy, of what it could mean to be an immigrant artist. In this dream, I am still me, nothing has changed, but I can write about literally anything other than immigration." Of course, the topics that Cornejo goes on to fantasize about addressing in her work—queer bison, the rehabilitation of police dogs, bees—are available to her, but the unstated constraint is what publishers want and expect from her.

She also describes the process of hardening her own boundaries about what she will and will not discuss at events and in interviews: "For the first few months, I would deflect the inevitable questions about immigration policy or my early years in Ecuador before my family came to America with my signature loquacious demurring. Then I had my partner, a professor who doesn't mince words, tell event organizers that I did not talk policy, particularly Donald Trump's zero-tolerance policy, and I did not talk about my own childhood separation." There is, of course, an irony in the fact that I—obviously a profound admirer of Cornejo—am including her work in a chapter about the very topic that most exhausts her. Yet I argue that what is most important to emphasize in her story—particularly as we grapple (as we will for a very long time) with the consequences of our government's brutality toward migrant children—is her insistence on the political origins of her trauma and her refusal to locate that trauma solely in the migration story of her parents. Like Zamora, Cornejo places the blame directly on the US government.

Remedio

The family separations that occurred under the Trump regime are horrifying to many people. They are particularly horrifying to me because they coincided with my own experience of parenthood: in the summer of 2018, as stories about family separation dominated the news, I became pregnant with twins, and the insomnia of late pregnancy and sleep deprivation of early parenthood were accompanied for me by endless doom scrolling as media report after media report surfaced about the brutal treatment of children who had been taken into US government custody. While the stories I read throughout 2018 and 2019 have had a particularly indelible effect on me, it has also become increasingly urgent for me to reflect on the fact that although family separations during the Trump regime were uniquely cruel (and illegal), family separation itself was not unique to the Trump administration and has been codified into US immigration law in troubling ways.

The first time I encountered family separation resulting from US immigration policy in a literary text, the author was not Latinx but Haitian American; I was an undergraduate literature student in the late 1990s. The text was Edwidge Danticat's novel *Breath, Eyes, Memory* (1995), a book that continues to shatter me every time I reread it. Although I do not offer an extended analysis of *Breath, Eyes, Memory* in this chapter (I am not a Danticat scholar and primarily read her work for pleasure), I could not have written this chapter without it. The novel is the story of Sophie Caco, born after her mother is raped by a paramilitary officer during the brutal dictatorship of Haiti's François "Papa Doc" Duvalier and raised by a maternal aunt and grandmother when her mother moves to the United States. Once reunited with her mother, Sophie is subjected to sexual abuse by her mother, who lives with unresolved trauma stemming from her rape and who ultimately dies by suicide. The novel is a gorgeous and wrenching exploration of what it means to be free in the aftermath of intergenerational trauma and gender-based violence. For Sophie, reunification with her mother is itself a source of trauma, not only because it means being subjected to abuse but also because it entails separation from her beloved aunt, whom Sophie regards as a maternal figure for the first twelve years of her life. But the novel also treats Sophie's mother with compassion, offering a nuanced portrait of a woman living with unresolved trauma in the wake of violence inflicted on her by a political regime led by a US-educated politician who came to be embraced by the US government (despite concerns about human rights) as an anti-communist ally. Furthermore, the novel demonstrates how an immigration policy that requires total separation from one's homeland severs both Sophie and her mother from their best source of support and thus negatively affects their wellbeing.

I consider Danticat to be an important theoretical guide for my analysis. Her book is particularly important to read now not only because of renewed attention to the ways in which anti-migrant violence at the US-Mexico border targets Haitians as well as Mexicans and Central Americans but also because of her insistence on representing migrants—including and especially those who both experience and inflict brutality—in their full complexity. In a moment when even progressive immigration rhetoric has become dominated by biocentric platitudes like "children belong with their parents," Danticat demonstrates the need to advocate for migrant wellbeing and family unification, while also refusing to gloss over the fact that family itself is often a site of trauma. Although it does not address our immediate political context, then, *Breath, Eyes, Memory* offers characters whose perspectives are necessary for understanding our current moment. And I believe that it is the fact that I have been sitting with the lessons that Danticat offers in that novel for more than two decades now that I was able to arrive at the particular readings I do of the works of Grande, Díaz, Zamora, and Cornejo.

In this chapter, I have examined texts suggesting that migrant justice and radical mental health require much more than the reunification and idealization of the nuclear family. Although none of the texts respond to the way immigration policy and rhetoric shifted in the Trump and post-Trump eras, all of them address the long-term impacts of family separation and refute the move to hold migrant parents solely responsible for its harms. Yet they do so without idealizing migrant parents. Radical health, as I have defined it in this book, entails both refusing the cultural imperative attached to normative health behaviors and advocating for access to health-sustaining support and resources. The texts I have examined in this chapter offer the beginnings of a vision of radical mental health, as they simultaneously refuse to ignore the psychic harms perpetuated within heteronormative family structures and also situate that harm within a wider geopolitical context.

Remedio

The Navigator

A year after the release of *Small Town Heroes*, the album that secured a place for Hurray for the Riff Raff in the American folk music canon, the band's singer-songwriter Alynda Mariposa Segarra wrote a column for *The Bluegrass Situation* denouncing the genre's lack of commitment to racial justice. "I feel so betrayed by the 'folk music' of today," they wrote. "Where is the outrage? Where is the love of justice and freedom for all? If you are too afraid to stand up for people who are marching in the streets saying 'STOP KILLING US' then you, friend, are not a folk singer" (Segarra 2015). Segarra calls on their contemporaries to embrace the genre's radical tradition during a resurgence of racial justice activism and decries the "cultural whitewashing" of folk music. Segarra's critique becomes even more pointed as they note their own ambivalent relationship to the current folk scene, describing how folk musicians of color are often tokenized: "As a folksinger, I have met with much appreciated critical acclaim this year. As a young Puerto Rican female, I have also been besieged by interviews questioning every part of my identity in the context of folk music. . . . When people of color are 'allowed' into the world of modern folk music we are held up as spokespeople. We are thought to be special, unlike the 'voiceless' others of our background."

As I confessed in chapter 3, I adore Alynda Mariposa Segarra and Hurray for the Riff Raff. Raised on my mother's Joan Baez and Joni Mitchell records before developing my own musical taste during a 1990s Riot Grrrl adolescence, I am quite a bit older than Segarra, but their particular blend of folk and feminist punk puts us on exactly the same musical wavelength.[1] From the moment I first heard Hurray for the Riff Raff's rendition of Mitchell's classic "River," from the 2013 covers album *My Dearest Darkest Neighbor*, I knew I had to find and listen to every song Segarra had ever sung.

But it isn't just the pull of Segarra's voice on my heart that makes their music so important to me. I found them when I was finishing my first book, my tenure book, which secured for me—a white woman—a professional presence in the field of Latinx studies. And the music of Segarra, a nonbinary Puerto Rican femme navigating the politics of race through and beyond a musical genre commandeered by whiteness, has traveled with me as I have sought ethical models for cross-racial aesthetic, affective, political, and intellectual engagement.

In 2017, when I was still in the early stages of writing *Radical Health*, Hurray for the Riff Raff dropped a new album, *The Navigator*, that escalated the challenge to folk music that Segarra launched in their 2015 essay. Previously hailed by *Pitchfork* as "one of the most compelling stylists in a folk revival full of suspicious acts either too beholden to tradition or too uncritical to make much of it" (Deusner 2014), Segarra called forth in *The Navigator* a more expansive folk music tradition than that most often highlighted in current folk revival, a racially diverse tradition they describe in their 2015 call-to-arms as "the warm embrace of singers like Odetta, Joan Baez, Lydia Mendoza, Harry Belafonte, Nina Simone, Buffy Sainte-Marie and Woody Guthrie." As music critic Ann Powers (2017) argues in her review of the album, *The Navigator* "repositions roots music as an anti-nostalgic tool: a truth-telling device."

The Navigator is a semi-autobiographical concept album, in which Segarra adopts an alter ego named Navita Milagros Negrón (Navi), who seeks to escape a constrained life in the Bronx before falling under the spell of a bruja and emerging forty years later to grapple with what she has lost.[2] The song "Pa'lante"—a tribute to the Young Lords—served as an anchor for both the album itself and the shows surrounding its release. Music critic Jenn Pelly (2022) describes it as a "masterpiece" that "triangulate[s] the past, present, and future . . . , traversing a continuum of historical struggle that is ongoing" and that demonstrates "not only what art is capable of but what it is for." At shows, Segarra frequently introduces the song by explaining the history and importance of the Young Lords; when audiences seem to tune out and talk through this introduction, they tell the crowd to "shut the fuck up and listen."[3] The song begins with Navi seeking survival among the ruins of late capitalism and ends with a recommitment to the Young Lords' revolutionary ideals that will lead the singer *pa'lante.*

The Navigator is also an enactment of the politics of radical health that I have elaborated throughout this book. The album is not explicitly "about" health but nonetheless insistently explores what it means to seek wellbeing in the midst of "exile, segregation and gentrification" (Powers 2017). In the opening track, "Living in the City," Navi orients the listener to life in a Bronx tenement—"fourteen floors of birthing and fourteen floors of dying" (Hurray for the Riff Raff 2017)—in which characters do whatever it takes to survive. Mariposa sings "love songs all in her dark apartment," while others succumb to overdoses and still others deliberately seek them out: "Gypsy bit the dust/You know the shit he had was poison/And now everybody wants just a taste of what we sold him" (Hurray for the Riff Raff 2017). Through its refusal to pathologize Mariposa's possibly depressive behavior or Gypsy's overdose, the song reflects the idea that—as the scholar Anna Kirkland proposes—"alternative ways of thinking about health are tied to necessary shifts in our thinking about concepts like risk, normality, vulnerability, accessibility, pleasure, and equality" (2010, 198). In the tracks that follow, Hurray for the Riff Raff goes on to invoke concerns of sexual health, emotional health, reproductive health, and environmental health, and specifically to elaborate the public health effects of displacement and gentrification; the official videos accompanying these songs were further inspired by the threats to public health posed by events following the album's release, including the Pulse nightclub shooting ("Hungry Ghost") and Hurricane Maria ("Pa'lante").[4] And, of course, the climactic song, "Pa'lante," specifically advocates a reevaluation of and recommitment to the activist project of the Young Lords, for whom health advocacy was a cornerstone of racial justice work. I have, therefore, taught *The Navigator* several times as a text that envisions radical health in both of the ways I define it in this book: as a repudiation of the stigma attached to unwellness in marginalized communities and as an exploration of the social conditions that can foster wellbeing within those communities.

The Navigator furthermore directly reinforces a secondary argument that infuses these pages: that art itself can intervene in the social conditions that impede the wellbeing of marginalized and disenfranchised people. The role of art as a form of personal solace surfaces in the opening track, with the aforementioned image of "Mariposa singing love songs all in her dark apartment." As the album—and Navi's journey—progresses, the role of art expands from a source of individualized comfort and pleasure to a political tool. In the song "Rican Beach," which takes place after Navi has awakened from the bruja's spell to find herself surveying the demise of the world she has known and loved, artists' abdication of their social responsibility is a direct cause of social collapse: "Now all the politicians, they just squawk their mouths/They say we'll build a wall to keep them out/ And all the poets were dying of a silence disease/So it happened quickly and with much ease." Here we see the consequences of the complacency for which Segarra calls out their fellow artists in their 2015 essay. Not all artists succumb to this "silence disease," however. The song "Pa'lante," in which Navi finds a path forward by looking to the past and embracing the wisdom of those who have preceded her, contains specific references to the artists who have served as Segarra's own navigators: Julia de Burgos, the Puerto Rican nationalist, feminist poet, and civil rights activist; Sylvia Rivera, the drag performer and trans liberation activist; and Pedro Pietri, cofounder of the Nuyorican Poets Café and member of the Young Lords. In this song, which represents the culmination of Navi's journey, not only is art inseparable from social justice struggle, but social justice is impossible to achieve without the imaginative work of art.

I evoke *The Navigator* in this final remedio not only as an instantiation of the arguments I have put forth throughout this book. I am also interested in the concept of the *navigator* that anchors the album. Segarra describes this concept:

> I wanted to say something about trying to escape who you are and where you come from: I loved the idea of "the navigator" because that means changing. What it means to me now is, who's driving the train? Do we know who's driving us? Do we know where we're going? Do we have a plan? Who's leading us? For me, that's been my inner guide or my intuition, but it also had to do with navigating identities and feeling like you live in the intersections of a lot of identities, like being Puerto Rican, being a woman, being queer, and also being from the Bronx. (Kaplan 2017)

In *The Navigator*, Navi seeks out her own navigator, an internal moral compass that guides her toward radical wellbeing not by moving away from her origins but by moving back into them. In this final remedio, then, I invoke my own navigator, exploring the intersections of my own journey, the personal histories that have brought me to this book.

I tell parts of these stories often in my teaching but less often in my research. As a white person with no apparent physical disabilities, it feels important to be clear with my students about my stakes in our work together, which are often different from theirs. Unlike me, many of my students are Latinx and have navigated the white supremacy of the Texas public education system with predominantly white teachers (including me). Like me, many have neurodevelopmental differences and unresolved trauma but no medical paperwork to access university-sanctioned accommodations. Like me, some are white students committed to anti-racist praxis and seeking ethical models for it. But as a white woman, discussing my social location in my research feels riskier; it brings up concerns about centering whiteness, about performative allyship, about empty gesturing, and I have largely avoided it until now.

I came to Latinx studies at the age of fourteen when my mother heard about Sandra Cisneros's *The House on Mango Street* (1984) and suggested I read it, thinking that it would help with what she called my "immigration issues." My parents had spent the previous three years working for a nongovernmental organization in Papua New Guinea, and our return to the United States had been difficult for me; it coincided with me hitting adolescence and questioning a lot of things about my childhood. My mother attributed my anger and insolence to our recent move (rather than to religious trauma or to a necessary critique of the white savior nonprofit industry that furnished our family's livelihood). As it turned out, *The House on Mango Street* did not have the effect my mother desired. I did not see myself or my life represented in its pages. The book prompted me to recognize that I needed to find an ethical place in the world that wasn't predicated on appropriating others' stories. And it suggested that literature might provide a way to grapple with my position in a racist social order—a position that (as I was beginning to sense but didn't yet have the critical tools to explain) was far less innocent than my parents had told me.

There *were* things about my life that I recognized in Cisneros's novel. Like the families in many of Cisneros's texts, mine had a lot of children and not much money, and we moved frequently: "What I remember most is moving a lot. Each time it seemed there'd be one more of us" (Cisneros [1984] 1991, 3). When we finally moved to a place where we didn't have to "share the yard with the people downstairs, or be careful not to make too much noise" (3), the house we settled in was "not the house we thought we'd get" (3). Like many of Cisneros's characters, I grew up in a mixed-class family that was usually broke, with a mother born into poverty and a father from the middle class. But unlike the parents of Cisneros's characters, mine were both college-educated and downwardly mobile, having undergone a religious conversion when I was eight years old that culminated in selling off or giving away their worldly possessions, joining the colonial apparatus (via a nonprofit that focused on international development), and moving us across the world. The protagonist of *Mango Street* has a father "who wakes up tired in the dark, who combs his hair with water, drinks his coffee, and is gone before we wake" (Cisneros [1984] 1991, 57). My parents were very different from that hardworking, responsible parent: they partied a lot, grew pot in the basement, got into conflicts with their supervisors, had a series of unplanned pregnancies followed by a rude awakening when Ronald Reagan dismantled what was left of the social safety net and food stamps weren't enough to feed us all, and eventually found Jesus (notably, *not* the kind of Jesus who requires renouncing psychoactive substances). I grew up with periods of food insecurity and no health insurance, with the heat getting cut off in the middle of winter, sleeping with siblings to stay warm, with secondhand clothes, with more siblings than my parents could support, without any money to inherit. But I also grew up certain I'd go to college, certain that if I made different choices than my parents had, I wouldn't live with economic precarity forever.

Years later, when I did make it to college and my love for *The House on Mango Street* led me to Nancy Saporta Sternbach's class on Latina women writers, I found more navigators. The text I remember most vividly from that class is Aurora Levins Morales's "Class Poem," which announces itself in the first line as "my poem in celebration of my middle class privilege" (Levins Morales and Morales 1986, 45). Levins Morales is the daughter of a poet and a university professor; these are not my parents' precise professions, but my parents also worked in a field (the nonprofit sector) that offered a lot of cultural capital without financial remuneration. Years before I came to appreciate Levins Morales as a disability justice activist, I encountered in her book *Getting Home Alive* (cowritten with her mother, Rosario Morales) the story of a young woman who grew up in an unconventional family, moving between rural Puerto Rico and the urban US mainland, highly educated but without generational wealth. The lines of "Class Poem" that hit me hardest as a college student and continue to hit me today are these:

And in case anyone here confuses the paraphernalia
with the thing itself
let me add that I lived with rats and termites
no carpet   no stereo   no TV
that the bath came in buckets and was heated on the stove
that I read by kerosene lamp and had Sears mail-order clothes
and that has nothing to do
with the fact of my privilege. (Levins Morales and Morales
    1986, 47)

With those lines, Levins Morales demanded from me an ethical stance in relation to my upbringing. Yes, I, too, had much of the "paraphernalia" of class oppression, and, no, my upbringing didn't contain the plot points of a typical middle-class story, but Levins Morales showed me the necessity of accounting honestly for *all* of the aspects of my story, the hard-fought struggles *and* the unearned advantages.

In November 2000, my younger sister fell and shattered a vertebra in her lower spine. She was nineteen, hanging out in the woods late at night with her boyfriend. They'd been drinking. She spent two months in the hospital in Atlanta, where I was living at the time. The rest of the family lived three hours away, where my younger brothers were in school and where my parents had to keep their jobs. They came and went as they could, and I saw my sister often during her rehabilitation.

    I wish that I remembered more about that hospital, especially now that there are a lot of things I can't ask my parents. Shepherd Center specializes in the treatment of spinal cord and brain injuries and offered what I now think of as classes on living with disabilities for newly disabled people and their loved ones. I attended as many of these as I could, some of which were very narrowly focused (how to change a catheter), and some of which felt like group therapy sessions. I often think that if I'd known about disability activism back then, or had a basic understanding of the US health care system, I would remember certain details better. (What was the co-pay for a two-month specialty hospital stay, and how did my parents afford it?

Was it only medical professionals we interacted with, or were there disability activists too? Is all the ableist messaging I recall from those classes a result of their entrenchment within the medical-industrial complex, the fact that they were filtered through my own ignorance and ableism, or a mix?) But the truth is that I was being flooded with secondary trauma, so who knows what I'd be able to pull from the fog of that time even if I had known to anticipate the questions I'd ask later.

Here's what I do remember: my sister *despised* the hospital that the rest of the family still speaks of reverently, the hospital that certainly saved her life and that likely offered my parents very generous financial assistance. She experienced her time there as a daily violation of her privacy and bodily autonomy. (Her family members were being taught *how to change her catheters*. Of course it was a violation.) The food was abhorrent to her. (I remember eating pudding from her tray and trying to ablesplain, much to her annoyance, that it "wasn't that bad.") There were constant disruptions, not to mention all the visitors my parents told her it was rude to turn away. I remember that facts were thrown at me in various meetings, and I remember not knowing what to do with them. *People with spinal cord injuries are more likely to develop substance abuse disorders. People with spinal cord injuries are more likely to end up in abusive relationships.* In short, I remember being presented, over and over, with my sister's bleak and terrifying future in a place where her lack of privacy and autonomy were taken for granted. And all of these memories are interspersed with the aftermath of a contested presidential election unfolding on the tiny television that hovered above her bed, where together we watched the Supreme Court install George W. Bush as president of the United States. No wonder my sister hated it there so fucking much.

Four years later, after I had moved away from Atlanta to go to graduate school, I attended a talk by Tobin Siebers. I went to the talk because I wanted the professor who organized it to join my dissertation committee, but I gained something I could not have imagined when I sat down in the lecture hall: the realization that there was nothing inevitable about the bleak future for my sister that had been presented to me in that hospital. That talk, the discovery of disability studies, changed my life. My first book, which I am now proud of in some ways and embarrassed by in others (does any writer ever feel anything but ambivalent about their own work?), is in many ways a reflection of what disability studies has given me. That book comes from a deep need to believe in disability as source of pride, as an identity to be joyfully claimed, as a form of political imagination that doesn't inevitably lead to failure or decay.

I still need to believe in all those things. And still do believe them.

But it is the *need* to believe in all those things that makes some parts of my first book sit uneasily with me now. I worry now about the extent to which my need for a recuperative crip politics may have led me to impose meanings on some of my texts. I don't know whether this is how my work reads to others, but I do know that while I was writing that book I was also imposing on my family a crip love story that wasn't fully true. I was recognizing in my family history the disabilities that we had lived with long before my sister's spinal cord injury—the mental illnesses, the stuttering, the asthma, the addictions, the cognitive differences. And I was learning from disability studies that these things did not have to be a source of trauma, a set of weapons we wielded against each other, a series of occasions for violence. They could be sites of joy and care and humor. But my family, although it had its moments of joy and care and humor, was much more committed to the cruelty than to the crip celebration.

The truth is that disability in my family has always been a source of shame, a topic to avoid, a target of abuse. The truth is that after my sister's accident the ableism that had always gone unexpressed in my family began to flourish in new and awful ways. After my sister's accident a story emerged in my family that my sister's disability was the only one in the family and also (contradictorily) that my sister was not really disabled. Ours, frankly, was an overcoming narrative. My sister was walking again. She had a healthy pregnancy and a gorgeous child. She lost touch with friends, but hadn't her friends been dubious influences anyway? And she didn't *want* to start a career after completing the college degree that got derailed by her accident; she wanted to be with her kid full-time, so it was good that she had a partner who ~~kept her from working~~ *took care of her* and ~~controlled~~ *supported* her.

It took me a long time to recognize that the crip narrative I wanted for my family wasn't real. One moment of awareness came after my sister, in the process of pursuing a neurodevelopmental diagnosis for her son, suggested to me that I have never been neurotypical. She presented facts and evidence from our childhood. She noted some of my stranger habits— which everyone in my family had always chalked up to the "quirkiness" that led me to become a professor—as elaborate strategies to compensate for executive function inconsistencies. *I'm not the only person in this family who is disabled*, she was telling me. When I started exploring the possibility of pursuing a diagnosis, the parental response was cold. "Did this whole disability studies thing make *you* decide to be disabled, too?" A much more dramatic shift occurred after my sister's marriage ended and the trauma she had managed for more than a decade began to manifest in new ways. When I supported (or, as my parents put it, *enabled*) her, my own family relationships shattered.

Radical Health was written while I was losing—and mourning—the possibility of a family story of crip joy. That loss has meant a painful realignment of my relationships with people I still—even in the face of distance, pain, and in at least one case total estrangement—love. It has also meant reckoning with the ways in which my family's ableism is deeply imbricated with our participation in and perpetuation of white supremacy.

As a white person working in ethnic studies, a disability scholar who presents to most people as able-bodyminded, I have long sought out the stories of scholars whose identities don't fully align with the subjects of their research, watching how narratives around allyship and alliance develop. Many of these stories hinge on race and class coalitions forged by growing up working-class/lower-middle-class or from interracial childhood bonds and disabled family members. I have these stories, too, but I want to tell a harder story: one about my own relationship with white supremacy and ableism, with ableist white supremacy. I believe that all white people have these stories and that we need to acknowledge and understand them if we are to be of any use in the struggle for racial justice. My parents had always been politically liberal and made it a point to raise me in racially heterogeneous environments, inside and outside the United States, but their liberalism also always had a heavy dose of Christian white benevolence mixed in: the idea that we were meant to make the world a better place, that our existence in the world as (white) Christian people was an inherently good thing, that we made the world a better place just by being ~~white~~ *Christian* in the world. Because the whiteness was always in parentheses, crossed out, or unspoken, it took me much longer than it should have to understand that liberal white benevolence is *also* white supremacy.

My sister's disability ruptured the narrative in a fundamental way. Suddenly a member of my family was not the *subject* of altruism but its object, someone targeted by others for acts of charity. ("Wow, you're actually really beautiful," said a stranger to my sister once, as she walked to a college classroom on forearm crutches. "Do people just expect me to be hideous?" she asked me when she told me this story later. "Do they think they are doing me a favor by talking to me?") Like the other disabilities in my family, my sister's disability had to be ignored, erased, and overcome as quickly as possible. This is what we told ourselves: my sister wasn't one of those disabled people we heard about in the hospital—the ones who developed substance abuse disorders and had abusive relationships, the ones who depended on government assistance and lived in poverty, the ones who experienced PTSD and other mental illnesses long after the traumatic accidents that caused their spinal cord injuries.

And when that narrative cracked, it was always her fault. If she noted that the family had been less than supportive during her time in the hospital, she was swiftly reminded that it was *her* drunken accident that inflicted stress and trauma and inconvenience on everyone else. When she needed more support than my parents offered during a contentious divorce from a partner who had economically controlled her for more than a decade, everyone was quick to insist they had never liked that guy anyway, had tried to warn her, had told her to leave sooner. "*I* didn't get her into that relationship; she needs to be accountable for her own choices," my father told me once in the middle of a fight about how I "enabled" her. The disabilities that flourish in my family are all stigmatized: substance use disorders, PTSD, the result of accidents while under the influence, mental illness, cognitive impairments. And instead of fighting the stigma, we hoard it and wield it against each other. Especially, we wield it against my sister, the most convenient target.[5]

But it isn't just our stigma we deny; it's also our privilege. My parents may have believed they were instilling in me a set of principles around racial equality, but conversations about race in my family always stopped short of acknowledging our relationship to white supremacy. The closest I've ever gotten my father even to admit to our whiteness was in a conversation about my youngest brother's addictions. At the time, my brother was in his early twenties and had been managing a substance use disorder for over a decade. "I hear about rising incarceration, and I really don't know how it is that he hasn't been in prison yet," my father said, in a moment of rare honesty between us. "He's white," I replied, "and white people in this country aren't the people they're building the cages for." "Maybe," my father said, and stood up and walked out of the room. Because my father—like me, like my brothers, like my nephew—*probably* has ADHD, it can be hard to tell whether he's ending a conversation because it's hit something close to home or because he's simply moved his attention somewhere else. I want to believe I made an important point and that my father heard it, but in truth I don't know.

In the introduction to *Black Disability Politics* (2022), published as I completed this book, Sami Schalk writes about her resistance to claiming disability identity as a fat, Black, queer woman:

> I just—despite over a decade of investment in disability studies—wasn't sure if I was allowed to really claim disability yet. I already have so many marginalized identities; it felt excessive. . . . What has prevented me from feeling that I can claim disability is the way my disabilities do not fit into the typical legal and medical models of disability and accommodations, the ways white disabled people especially have been dismissive of my understanding of how racism, sexism, homophobia, classism, and fatphobia have materially created, sustained, and exacerbated my disabilities. I cannot get on board with approaches to disability that do not understand it as inherently, inextricably tied to racism and other oppressions. I cannot and will not promote a disability-first or disability-pride-only analysis. (2)

Schalk's honesty in writing about the difficulty of naming herself as disabled resonates deeply with me. Which is *not* to say that I understand our situations as analogous: Although Schalk and I share the fact that we both became disability scholars before we identified as disabled people, our stories of claiming disability clearly diverge. If for Schalk, "racism, sexism, homophobia, classism, and fatphobia" have "created, sustained, and exacerbated" her disabilities, in my own case many of these same ideologies have provided support, making it unnecessary or even too much trouble to seek accommodations and formal diagnoses. But because I—like Schalk—understand disability as "inherently, inextricably tied to racism and other oppressions," I have also hesitated to describe myself as disabled. As a white person in particular, I am wary of how claims to disability identity can occlude the participation of white people in systems of oppression. Alison Kafer and Eunjung Kim remind us that "some disabled people are more marginalized than others" and that "some disabled people may benefit from the conditions that hinder others" (2017, 128). Yet too often, white disability scholars have been complicit with a narrative in which "disability is considered to 'trump' race, or disabled people are understood as the 'most discriminated against' category" (127). Although my first book is invested in the political potential of disability identity, I now emphasize its dangers—the dangers, in particular, of how the intersection of whiteness with what Schalk calls a "disability-first or disability-pride-only analysis" can erase and appropriate racial oppression.

As *Radical Health* began to form as a book in my mind, it therefore became important for me to move away from examining disability identity and to focus instead on what disability and critical ethnic studies teach us about the cultural and political implications of health stigma. As I have noted, health stigma has been a powerful weapon in my family, something we brandish to deny each other support and care, something we exert to thwart each other's wellbeing. This book's focus on health stigma—and on writers and artists who offer tools for challenging its wide-ranging and damaging effects—is a direct result of that experience. Because the abusive deployment of health stigma had become so familiar to me on an intimate, personal level in the years since my sister's accident, it was immediately recognizable (and immediately recognizable as violent) when I saw it happening on a national level in the years just before I began to conceptualize and write this book (2009–2016). Specifically, as the crafting and then the passage of the Affordable Care Act became a focus of national conversations, the political discourse I was suddenly hearing everywhere—about *people who don't take care of themselves* and *people expecting the government to take care of them*—recalled for me the conversations in my own family about how *she brings this on herself*. In a recent essay describing her own experience as a witness to ableist domestic violence, Jina B. Kim (2019) elaborates how the public devaluation of disabled people works in tandem with intimate abuse:

> As good feminists, many of us know that it is not just individual acts of physical and sexual assault that constitute rape culture, but also a victim-blaming and sense of entitlement to the bodies of others. Fewer of us know that ableism—which involves both active discrimination against disabled people *and also* a shared cultural contempt for vulnerability, care labor, and people's physical/emotional needs—also enables certain forms of abuse to flourish, allowing care to become its own form of violence. (195)

Even as I found myself enraged and aggrieved in a deeply personal way by pundits arguing about who "deserved" health care and who didn't, my emotional response often failing to distinguish the politicians who blamed communities for their health outcomes from my parents blaming my sister for her physical and emotional collapses, intellectually I did recognize a crucial difference between the national conversations and those taking place within my family. While the familial conversation and the national conversation bore undeniable similarities, there was another layer to the national conversation: the discourse of health stigma and blame within my white family has circulated as ableist *interpersonal* violence, but the discourse of health stigma and blame within my white supremacist nation has circulated as ableist *racial* violence.[6]

To argue that debates about who should receive health care in the United States are manifestations of racial violence and white supremacy is not, I hasten to add, to argue that all white people benefit from them in the same way. As scholars of whiteness (and critical race studies in general) regularly point out, the institution of whiteness does not necessarily confer on all white people the same benefits. In perhaps the most relevant of these studies for my project in *Radical Health*—a book aptly titled *Dying of Whiteness*—Jonathan M. Metzl examines the decline in white health and life expectancy that occurred in red states immediately after Donald Trump's rise to power.[7] He argues: "This is because white America's investment in maintaining an imagined place atop a racial hierarchy—that is, an investment in a sense of whiteness—ironically harms the aggregate well-being of US whites as a demographic group, thereby making whiteness itself a negative health indicator" (2019, 9). My family almost seems like a case study for Metzl's study, given the ways in which we routinely use against each other the very same health stigma that targets each of us, but for one detail: Metzl's focus on how and why "white Americans . . . support right-wing politicians and policies, even when these policies actually harm white Americans at growing rates" (9). My family does not support right-wing politicians, but it is, nonetheless, invested in its "imagined place atop a racial hierarchy." Where my own white lived experience complicates Metzl's argument, then, is where it pushes me to insist that white supremacy is not the exclusive purview of white people identified with the political right in this country; white supremacy can pervade and motivate the political left as well. For this insight I draw from the work of cultural studies scholar Lee Bebout, whose book *Whiteness on the Border* elaborates how "U.S. nationalism and the U.S. racial imagination function through anti-Mexican [and, I would add, anti-Latinx] forms of racialization" (2016, 5). Bebout does not limit his analysis to cultural artifacts associated with a right-wing political agenda and even explicitly considers the racializing effects found in the purportedly "positive" representations of cultural objects oriented around white *desire* for Mexican people. Like Bebout, I believe it is important to consider that although white people are not universally the *beneficiaries* of white supremacy, we are all likely to be its *participants* at some point in our lives, even when acting out of purported love and beneficence, unless (and even if) we develop deliberate and intentional frameworks for consistently acting—and even structuring our lives—against it.

This book, then, is one of my deliberate and intentional efforts against white supremacy, a white supremacy of which I nevertheless cannot fully absolve myself, a white supremacy whose insidious and constant presence requires my continuous vigilance. However, although the book began because I recognized in the public discourse about a national health care plan the same abusive impulse that undergirded my family's acts of health shaming, and because my recognition of the white supremacist impulses within my family's ableism led me to understand how that health shaming on a national level functioned in the service of a racializing national discourse, that is not where it has ended.

Instead of taking the approach of Metzl and Bebout, who base their analyses in ethnographic research and cultural criticism focused on white communities and artists, I have instead focused my analysis on Latinx writers and artists whose work offers for me an essential corrective to the racializing effects of health stigma. There are two fundamental reasons for this choice. One is practical: I was trained as a cultural critic working in the field of Latinx studies; this is the aesthetic archive I know best. The other is emotional: the texts I write about in this book are those that sustained me through the rage and grief that initially propelled it. Not only have they sustained me, they have taught me. It is through deep engagement with these texts that I have learned that another understanding of health and wellbeing is possible. I understand these texts as necessary for my liberation, for my sister's liberation—which is not to say that I understand these texts as having been created *for* my liberation, or for my sister's. I do, however, believe that these texts have helped me to see white supremacy itself as a health threat and have put me on a path of working to eradicate it. The journalist Linda Villarosa, whose recent book *Under the Skin* argues that racism itself must be studied as the key factor leading to the unequal health outcomes experienced by Black Americans and other people of color in the United States, also argues that racism is not a problem for people of color alone to solve: racism, she writes, "is the American problem in need of an American solution" (2022, 21). The texts I write about in this book are some of the texts that have helped point me toward a solution, the texts that have offered me a vision of the world I want to work for and shown me what I need to do to help make it.

In their open letter to the folk music community, Segarra (2015) urges their fellow musicians to join the struggle for racial justice: "You do not have to have the same skin to feel that pain. . . . Even If you are not personally affected by the oppression that is killing black and brown people, you still have a place in this revolution." On its surface these words can be read as naive, a too-easy call-in. But as I've already demonstrated, I'm a Segarra fangirl, so I always choose the generous reading when it comes to their work. I don't read these words as an invitation for me to claim "the same pain" that I see reflected in the work of the artists and writers who inspired this book. Instead, I see in their work the blueprints for a social world that will create less pain for *all of us.* I read Segarra's words as an exhortation to do the work, to reimagine coalition, to be held accountable. I find this call as well in each of the texts I examine in *Radical Health.* This book is not my only effort to join the struggle for health justice that I see taking place in the texts I've examined here, but it is one effort, an effort that I hope you find meaningful. I hope this book helps to make more work possible, just as the literature and performance art and music I write about in these pages have made possible the work I seek to do in the world.

NOTES

INTRODUCTION: RADICAL HEALTH/RADICAL UNWELLNESS

1   Mae M. Ngai argues that during the period following the Johnson-Reed
    Act of 1924, "restrictive immigration laws produced new categories of
    racial difference" (2004, 34–35). More specifically, she notes that during
    the late 1920s, the "actual and imagined association of Mexican with illegal
    immigration was part of an emergent Mexican 'race problem,' which also
    witnessed the application of Jim Crow segregation to Mexicans in the
    Southwest, especially in Texas, and, at the federal level, the creation of
    'Mexican' as a separate racial category in the census" (36). In her history
    of the United States Border Patrol (established by the Johnson-Reed Act),
    Kelly Lytle Hernandez portrays immigration enforcement as "a site of
    racialization and inequity in the United States" (2010, 3). Building on these
    points, Natalia Molina's history of Mexican immigration to the United
    States between 1924 and 1965 bears the title *How Race Is Made in America*;
    she forcefully argues that "if we are to understand why we think about race
    and citizenship the way we do, we must thoroughly examine immigra-
    tion laws and practices because they structure and lend meaning to these
    concepts" (2014, 11). Meanwhile, more recent works by Monica Muñoz
    Martinez and Beth Lew-Williams examine the role of racial violence in

constructing particular groups of people as perpetually foreign; Martinez portrays anti-Mexican violence in early twentieth-century South Texas as "a past that bleeds into the present, a suppression that continues to shape our future" (2018, 10), while Lew-Williams (2018) elaborates how anti-Chinese violence gave rise to immigration restrictions like the 1882 Chinese Exclusion Act, even as such laws fomented further violence.

2 *Bodymind* is a term that I first encountered in the work of Margaret Price, who explains: "Because mental and physical processes not only affect each other but also give rise to each other—that is, because they tend to act as one, even though they are conventionally understood as two—it makes more sense to refer to them together, in a single term" (2015, 269). Expanding on Price's work, Sami Schalk highlights the term's particular utility for discussing experiences of racialized disability, noting that the term "can help highlight the relationship of nonphysical experiences of oppression—psychic stress—and overall wellbeing" (2018, 6).

3 Consider, for instance, Lennard Davis's famous and widely cited critique of the "kill-or-cure" ending of many disability narratives: "The alterity presented by disability is shocking to the liberal, ableist sensibility, and so narratives involving disability always yearn for the cure, the neutralizing of the disability" (2002, 99). The implication here is that a "yearn for the cure" always and only derives from ableist impulses.

4 Schalk and Kim critique the "cursory or comparative inclusion of race" (2020, 35) in much disability scholarship, a critique supported by the fact that the brief history recounted here is virtually unknown in disability studies. As one noteworthy example, the story of Isabel González is completely absent from the definitive history of disability and immigration, Douglas C. Baynton's *Defectives in the Land*, despite Baynton's emphasis on "the intersections between race and disability in immigration law" (2016, 6), despite the importance of the story to the construction of race in the twentieth-century United States, and despite the explicit role of visible physical difference in González's detention.

5 For more on the politics of work and care as related to both welfare reform and the ADA, see Frye 2016 and J. B. Kim 2021.

6 Laura Briggs writes: "The welfare reform discussion that began under Reagan provided the cultural cover to initiate this massive economic restructuring, and it involved a deliberate, policy-driven shift in political power away from unions, people of color, and women, and to corporations and the wealthy. It was mobilized in ways that particularly affected women and people of color and traded on negative stereotypes of those groups to effect its changes while not seeming callous. The poor, it told us, were responsible for their own poverty through their bad choices" (2017, 73–74).

7 For a report of Chaffetz's comments, see Shelbourne 2017. For an analysis of how the cost of a new iPhone in 2017 actually compared to the average cost

of health care at that time (and, thus, for a full account of the dishonesty and callousness of Chaffetz's remarks), see Ingraham 2017.

8 On this point, Anna Kirkland and Diana Bowman coedited a special issue of the *Journal of Health Policy, Politics and Law*, entitled "The Law and Politics of Workplace Wellness," inspired by the ACA's changes to rules governing workplace wellness programs, notably its creation of an exception to the nondiscrimination provisions of the Health Insurance Portability and Accountability Act (HIPAA). This special issue, and particularly Kirkland's contribution, is not extensively cited here but catalyzed my thinking as I began to conceptualize this book. See Kirkland 2014.

9 Gordon (2013) cites the law's reliance on employer-based insurance and states' willingness to expand Medicaid, also major flaws.

10 The anthropologist Jonathan Xavier Inda terms this the "necropolitics of uncare" (2020, 700). Inda develops the term through an analysis of preventable deaths, often resulting from the withholding of medical care, of immigrants in US Immigration and Customs Enforcement (ICE) detention; he argues that such immigrants "are allowed to perish in the name of protecting and nurturing the life of the national population—making it clear that migrant lives do not matter" (703). Although the situations that inspire Inda's term are particularly horrific, I would argue that the term also applies to more mundane, routinized instances in which racialized populations are either outright denied treatment or given substandard care.

11 The concept *healthism* is also usefully developed in the work of Julie Guthman (2011) and Anna Kirkland (2011).

12 I include addiction on this list despite studies showing that drug use is more prevalent in white communities than in communities of color, and despite the concentration of a widely publicized opioid addiction crisis in rural white communities as I write, because of evidence suggesting that addiction is more likely to be treated as a health problem for white people experiencing it and more likely to be criminalized for people of color experiencing it. In this sense, even if addiction is not more *prevalent* in communities of color, its effects are still more devastating.

13 In this regard, it is useful to contrast Barack and Michelle Obama to Bill and Hillary Clinton, who spearheaded an effort during the 1990s to create a national health care system that failed spectacularly. Bill Clinton (who famously became a vegan after leaving the presidency) was often photographed eating hamburgers on the campaign trail, and his dietary habits were a target of satire. Hillary Clinton, appointed to chair the task force that created the Clinton health care plan, was skewered by the right for overreaching what was considered to be the role of the First Lady (devotion to a charitable cause without ambition to create policy). For more substantial analysis of Michelle Obama's *Let's Move!* campaign, see Cowing 2020 and Kulbaga and Spencer 2017.

14 Bonilla-Silva's term for this racial ideology is *color-blind racism*. Although I find Bonilla-Silva's insights absolutely indispensable, I choose not to employ this term in order to heed the warnings of disability scholars about the problems with using bodily and sensory impairments as metaphors for social problems.

15 I am inspired by scholars who have expanded Charon's approach. Notably, Phillip J. Barrish proposes that "we who study intersections of literature and medicine should devote more sustained attention to literary engagements with health care as a system: a complex, often fragmented set of financial models, institutions, government policies, and personnel whose roles range well beyond patient and care provider" (2016, 106). Olivia Banner proposes reading not for the illness narrative but for "the politics of illness" (2016, 32), advocating a "move away from the current emphasis on individuals learning to behave better and instead toward individuals understanding how institutions and structures condition that behavior" (45). And Charon's colleagues at Columbia, Yoshiko Iwai, Zahra H. Khan, and Sayantani DasGupta, propose a revision of narrative medicine as abolition medicine, which aims "to renarrate and re-envision justice, healing, activism, and collectivity" (2020, 159).

16 For instance, I am not interested in the argument that *Latinx* constitutes a form of linguistic imperialism simply because it seeks to subvert the grammatical gender of the Spanish language; as a teacher, I aspire to a pedagogy that eschews valuations of "correct" grammar in any language, so it doesn't make sense to import such valuations into my scholarship. However, I do have some affinity for the argument (made by Richard T. Rodríguez and others) that *Latinx,* which arises out of a desire to include nonbinary people who don't identify with either the *A* or the *O* in *Latina/o,* actually has the opposite effect when used "for the express purpose of shorthand (i.e., making things easier with the singular X rather than form an unwieldy term consisting of too many pronouns)" (Rodríguez 2017, 205–6).

1. UNPROTECTED TEXTS

1 This is not to argue that people should not take precautions against the transmission of STDs. It is to acknowledge that "un/protected" sex is a category that shifts in meaning with advances in knowledge about HIV transmission and the availability of new drug therapies, especially pre-exposure prophylaxis (PrEP) drugs. Condom use, serosorting, oral and manual sex, preventative drugs, and strategic positioning are all HIV prevention strategies with varying degrees of availability, cost, effectiveness, and risk—and given the vagueness of the term, all could be described as "protected" or "unprotected." My point, then, is that attaching stigma and shame to "unprotected" sex, especially when the meaning of the term is so imprecise, is not an effective public health measure. As Paula A. Treichler argues: "AIDS

is to be a fundamental force of twentieth-century life, and no barrier in the world can make us 'safe' from its complex material realities" (1999, 40).

2   The Center for HIV Law and Policy (2022) offers a comprehensive and deeply sobering guide to HIV-positive criminal statutes.

3   This section is based on an earlier essay of mine that contains extended readings of additional pieces from *City of God*; see Minich 2017.

4   Thankfully, this is less and less true. Notable recent or forthcoming analyses of Cuadros's work include Marissa K. López's *Racial Immanence: Chicanx Bodies beyond Representation* (2019), Pablo Alvarez's dispatch contribution to *AIDS and the Distribution of Crises* (Cheng, Juhasz, and Shahani 2020), and Joshua Javier Guzmán's forthcoming book *Dissatisfactions: Queer Chicano Style Politics*.

5   Aztlán, believed to be the original homeland of the Mexica/Aztec people and located in the present-day US Southwest, is the enduring ideological construct of Chicanx cultural nationalism. I engage substantially with Aztlán in my first book (Minich 2014) and don't repeat that engagement here. Aztlán is usually spelled with an accent mark; however, Cuadros writes "Aztlan" without the accent mark, and I follow this practice when quoting him. (I otherwise use the accent mark.)

6   The construction of the Los Angeles Freeway (and in particular the East Los Angeles Interchange, completed in the 1960s) destroyed many of Los Angeles's multiethnic communities. Eric Avila characterizes it as "wreaking havoc on the city's heterosocial spaces and accelerating the trend to postwar agglomeration of racially segregated communities" (2004, 181). Among aesthetic representations, the work of Helena María Viramontes—including both the novel *Their Dogs Came with Them* (2007) and the short story "Neighbors" (1985)—offers a particularly memorable depiction of this havoc.

7   In an earlier essay on Cuadros, I examine another representation of a family that exceeds heteronormative kinship structures in the short story "Reynaldo," also in *City of God*; see Minich 2017.

8   Dosed in combination with other antiretroviral therapies, AZT remains an important component of HAART.

9   The "morally censorious and fear-mongering" (Tomso 2004, 99) *Rolling Stone* article that introduced the phrase *bug chasing* into mainstream discourse, Gregory Freeman's "In Search of Death" (2003), portrays the practice as a form of self-harm, exaggerates its occurrence, and pathologizes it. Freeman exclusively interviews bug chasers and a behavioral psychiatrist, largely ignoring the voices of seropositive men (except for those identifying as reformed bug chasers). Furthermore, although Freeman does not explicitly identify the races of the men he interviews, he uses the pseudonym Carlos for the bug chaser most prominently featured in the article, thus implicitly racializing the practice.

10 Octavio R. González importantly identifies the bug chaser as "an apocryphal figure in our contemporary cultural landscape" (2010, 87) who

exists discursively to reinforce "the normative logic of . . . AIDS Inc." (97); his analysis of this figure notes that it can "radically challenge the assimilation of 'gay' as an 'all-but-hetero' normative collective identity (the contemporary homonormativity of marriage, adoption, and so on)" (106). I am compelled by González's analysis and want to distinguish my own analysis from the representations González critiques: I don't think Cuadros is invoking the figure of the HIV-negative man seeking sex with an HIV-positive partner in order to secure a "normative collective identity"; rather, I think Cuadros is illustrating the vulnerability of HIV-positive people in sexual encounters with HIV-negative people. Such individuals are, as Decena (2008) points out, subjected to regimes of compulsory disclosure but unprotected from sexual violence.

11 Louise Hay was a motivational speaker known for her belief that people become ill due to their lack of self-love; she is remembered for exploiting HIV/AIDS in her rise to prominence.

12 It is worth reiterating that the story was written decades before the availability of smartphones and transit apps.

13 Given that many of Cuadros's protagonists struggle with internalized racism and express preferences for white lovers (a fact often emphasized by critics), I do not completely discount the possibility that there is a racial basis for the narrator's refusal of this advance. Nonetheless, given the events of the story, it is possible that the narrator is too tired or hungover to respond, or that after the violence of the previous night he is not aroused. Furthermore, as I will discuss in the following section, and as I elaborate at even greater length in my previous essay on *City of God* (Minich 2017), Cuadros does discuss erotic attachments to men of color in the book, a fact that critics often ignore.

14 In her study of ACT UP/LA, Benita Roth identifies Silver Lake as the neighborhood where the Mattachine Society was founded in 1950 and as "a place where lesbians and gays worked in coalition with that area's working-class Latino families" during the 1990s (2017, 13).

15 "Johnson's Market" likely refers to the JonSon's Market chain, a onetime East LA institution whose stores have since been bought out by other minimarket chains.

16 Ralph E. Rodriguez has suggested to me that my reading of this poem fails to adequately account for the cynicism with which Cuadros's speaker recounts their hands lingering on his neck in the first stanza and the bitterness with which he expresses a desire to tell them he loves them in the third. I am grateful to Rodriguez for pointing this out, and after considering this objection, I concede that I may have misread the poem (and, thus, have probably been too gentle in my assessment of likely sexual assailants), but I remain attached to my reading and have left it as is. Perhaps this is only because I previously published this interpretation, but I think there's actually something deeper here: that my potential misreading actually

speaks to the ways in which being simultaneously bullied and aroused is an uncomfortable part of my own sexual history, a part of my sexual history that is partly why I am so emotionally drawn to Cuadros's work. To put it bluntly, my sexual attractions and commitments have not always been deemed by others (or myself) as emotionally "healthy," and I love Cuadros for offering me a way to explore the confusing experience of how sexual pleasure and sexual violence can intermingle (an experience that has also, in many ways, motivated my analysis in chapter 3 of this book).

17   *Sexile* was published by the Institute for Gay Men's Health, a partnership of the Gay Men's Health Crisis (GMHC) and AIDS Project Los Angeles (APLA).

18   Sandoval-Sánchez's work on abjection is also a touchstone for the performance critic Leticia Alvarado, whose work figures prominently in other sections of this book.

19   It is worth noting that this disparagement campaign, explicitly named by Peña, is part of a broader cultural investment in heteropatriarchy that characterized the early decades of the Cuban Revolution; this broader cultural tendency has been documented in numerous cultural artifacts, with the memoir *Antes que anochezca* (1992), written by fellow queer Mariel exile Reinaldo Arenas, serving as one well-known and detailed account.

20   It is also worth noting here that while Vázquez's individual account depicts her accessing gender-affirming health care after relocating from Cuba to the United States, health care in Cuba is generally much more equitably available; this is often attributed to the revolution, but the historian Daniel A. Rodríguez has recently argued that the Cuban state's commitment to a "right to health for all Cubans" (2020, 18) actually dates back much earlier, to independence.

21   Vázquez herself, in an oral history narrative published a decade after *Sexile*, describes her own approach to HIV/AIDS prevention work: "I had never liked going to places where people were looking for cock and telling them, 'Hold on, I wanna talk to you about condoms.' I wanted to do something that would please me" (2015, 216).

22   Rendell and Diedrich do not cite Saidiya Hartman, whose critique of empathy in *Scenes of Subjection* (1997) and "Venus in Two Acts" (2008) urges us to consider who actually benefits from "empathetic" accounts that tell others' stories. Given Campo's social positioning vis-à-vis his patients, however, I would argue that Hartman's critique absolutely has purchase here.

23   Campo's most recent collection, *Comfort Measures Only: New and Selected Poems, 1994–2016* (2018), includes a number of his poems about HIV/AIDS among the collected earlier poems but none solely about the virus in the section devoted to new poetry.

24   When it was first published in the scholarly *Journal of Medical Humanities*, the poem was titled "Wednesday HIV Clinic" (Campo 2013b); it was subsequently retitled for *Alternative Medicine*.

25 Later revealed as Timothy Ray Brown, the Berlin patient made headlines in 2008 as the first person to be cured of HIV.

26 Although Wald vociferously critiques the narratives that vilify disease carriers like Mary Mallon and Gaëtan Dugas, her book was published eight years before genetic sequencing of virus samples definitively cleared Dugas's name; see Doucleff 2016.

2. SUGAR, SHAME, LOVE

1 In presenting material from this chapter to various audiences over the years, I have often been asked why I do not discuss the work of Gloria Anzaldúa, who wrote movingly of her experience with diabetes in the essay "now let us shift . . ." from her final coedited anthology, *This Bridge We Call Home* (2002). The primary reason for this choice is that Anzaldúa's engagements with illness have received extensive critical attention from other scholars, and so I prefer to recommend that readers consult the work of Rebeca L. Hey-Colón (2022), Andrea J. Pitts (2021), Amanda Ellis (2021), Amelia M. L. Montes (2016), and Suzanne Bost (2010, 2015).

2 As of this writing, there is no definitive number for the death toll for Hurricane Maria. For months after the storm, the official count was 64; in August 2018, former governor Ricardo Roselló was finally forced by the release of a study from George Washington University to revise the official death toll to 2,975. However, other studies—including an earlier Harvard study that specifically looked at the consequences of delayed medical care—have placed the number above 4,000; see Fink 2018. For more information on the role of Puerto Rico's journalists in this debate, see Minet 2019. For a historical analysis of the racialized neglect of diabetic people affected by natural disasters, see Richard M. Mizelle Jr.'s (2020) stunning work on the impact of Hurricane Katrina on diabetic residents of the Gulf Coast. Additionally, I wish to acknowledge here my gratitude to Kayla Shearer for reminding me that insulin dependence, while a defining characteristic of type 1 diabetes, is not universal among type 2 diabetics. However, because insulin dependence tends to present in type 2 diabetics whose conditions have received less consistent treatment, it is important to remember that the populations of both Puerto Rico and coastal Texas include high numbers of insulin-dependent type 2 diabetics.

3 Throughout this chapter, I primarily cite Berlant's 2007 article titled "Slow Death (Sovereignty, Obesity, Lateral Agency)," which appeared in the journal *Critical Inquiry*; a later version of the article appeared as a chapter in Berlant's 2011 book *Cruel Optimism*, but the article remains widely cited on its own (and is more accessible to readers without academic library privileges; as of this writing a PDF of the article is freely available online).

4 Hatch's notion of biomedical individualism also aligns nicely with Robert Crawford's notion of healthism, discussed in the introduction. I use Hatch's terminology in this chapter because he derives his term specifically from a discussion of race and metabolic disease.

5 In the final chapter of this book, I engage extensively with recent work by La Marr Jurelle Bruce on racialized madness, work that interrogates how "reason and rationality are believed essential for achieving modern personhood, joining civil society, and participating in liberal politics" even as they are also deeply entangled "with misogynist, colonialist, ableist, antiblack, and other pernicious ideologies" (2021, 4). My proposal that certain kinds of health practices associated with poverty, particularly around nutrition, might be understood as *rational* may seem to counter the stances I take elsewhere in this book questioning the use of rationality as a measure of social value. I acknowledge this tension. Bruce asserts that madness "often functions as a disparaging descriptor for any mundane phenomenon perceived to be odd and undesirable," including an "unconventional hairstyle, unpopular political opinion, physical tic, indecipherable utterance, eccentric outfit, dramatic flouting of etiquette, apathy toward money and wealth, or experience of spiritual ecstasy" (2021, 8). I would argue that eating a diet unsanctioned by contemporary nutritionists certainly falls into this category, and that Berlant—while not using the words *mad* or *crazy* to describe the people who consume such diets—nonetheless ascribes to them what Bruce calls "an *unruliness of will* that resists and unsettles reigning regimes of the normal" (2021, 8; original emphasis). My point here is not to affirm the social value of rationality but simply to note that one way the social value of rationality accumulates is through its systemic denial to populations already devalued by race and class ideologies.

6 Nixon himself is clear that climate change is only one form of slow violence; indeed, to illustrate the concept, he uses the example of intimate partner violence. Additionally, as the work of Richard M. Mizelle Jr. (2020) on the intersections of chronic disease and environmental disasters has demonstrated, climate change is not entirely irrelevant to this discussion, although not my focus here.

7 The name derives from a line Sotomayor has used in a number of her speeches, one of which was reprinted in the *Berkeley La Raza Law Journal*, that prompted vociferous debate during her 2009 confirmation hearings: "I would hope that a wise Latina woman with the richness of her experiences would more often than not reach a better conclusion than a white male who hasn't lived that life" (Sotomayor 2002, 92). While opponents of Sotomayor's confirmation used the line to question her impartiality, supporters seized on it, gleefully printing mugs and T-shirts with the words *wise Latina.*

8 For instance, in *My Beloved World*, she boasts of "racking up convictions" (2013, 204) when describing her time as a prosecutor, while *Turning Pages*

includes several didactic passages about the importance of laws that led me to cringe when I read the book to my own children.

9 As this book goes to production (February 2023), the Supreme Court has upheld the ACA, but it continues to face challenges in court.

10 Historian Richard M. Mizelle Jr. reminds us that the stigma attached to type 2 diabetes is "misguided," noting that both types are "the result of multiple, overlapping genetic, social, cultural, and environmental determinants" (2020, 123).

11 In this sense, Sotomayor provides a point of contrast to another Latina public figure with type 1 diabetes: Robin Arzón, vice president of fitness programming for Peloton, whose public statements about the disease often replicate what disability scholars call a "supercrip" narrative: "I want to normalize the idea that superheroes are real . . . and I want folks to be the living embodiment of real life superheroes," she stated in a recent interview (Kenney 2021).

12 It is not the central purpose of this chapter, so I will not elaborate on this point, but I do love this passage for its critique of heteronormativity: the ways in which Sotomayor describes herself as "a mannequin" trapped in a ritual that is not built to accommodate her nonnormative body. On this point, it is also worth noting that the marriage ends in divorce and that at the end of the book, Sotomayor describes her friendships (not one life partner) as the sustaining force of her life, noting that "families can be made in other ways" (2013, 235).

13 For instance, the *Washington Post* reported that the price of Humalog insulin increased by 700 percent (adjusted for inflation) in the two decades between 1996 and 2016. This statistic was included in an article about controversies surrounding Donald Trump's nominee to head the Department of Health and Human Services, Alex Azar (whose offensive remarks about meatpacking workers affected by COVID-19 are discussed in the introduction to this book). During Azar's five years as an executive at Eli Lilly, the company that sells Humalog insulin, its price more than doubled, eventually prompting a class-action lawsuit (C. Johnson 2017). Eli Lilly and its insulin pricing were also directly targeted in the chaos that ensued at Twitter after Elon Musk's 2022 acquisition of the company and short-lived launch of Twitter Blue, a paid program that briefly enabled ordinary people to impersonate corporations and celebrities; after a user impersonating Eli Lilly tweeted that the company would provide free insulin, the company's stock fell by more than 5 percent (Mac et al. 2022).

14 See Luis 2014 and Lomas 2014a, 2014b on these themes in Laviera's work.

15 "I transitioned from poetry to plays because I typed with two fingers. When I lost my eyesight I couldn't type because I never learned how . . . I adapted to working with people who would hear my voice and type, from voice to finger. And this transition made it easier for me to develop characters or

do other kinds of writing that I used to not like more than poetry because poetry is more personal." My translation.

16 On the oral aesthetics of Laviera's poetry, see Alvarez 2006 and E. López 2014; Glenn Martínez (2014) also offers a useful interpretation of "Word."

17 "I never paid attention to all these things . . . total negligence." My translation.

18 For instance, I saw a 2015 production directed by Rudy Ramirez for Teatro Vivo in Austin, Texas, in which the piece was performed by three actresses.

19 For more on the problems of Ensler's piece, especially its transmisogyny, see Hall 2005.

20 In the monologue titled "Noticias," which consists of "facts gathered from our hometown newspaper, the San Antonio *Express-News*," the authors include a headline stating that "S.A. ranks as nation's fattest city on fed list . . . study shows 31.1% of Alamo City residents are obese" (Grise and Mayorga 2014, 65). Google searches easily turn up lists showing San Antonio in the top five most obese cities, but most of these lists are from the early 2000s. The most recent list I could find while writing this chapter listed San Antonio as number nineteen, with the McAllen-Edinburg-Mission metro area (in the region discussed at the beginning of this chapter, the Valley) taking the number-one spot (Menchaca 2019).

21 Building on the research published in peer-reviewed journals like the study cited here, Fielding-Singh has also recently published a compelling book aimed for a general readership arguing that instead of "heaping more responsibility and judgement onto parents' plates for what goes in kids' bodies, we can begin to regard kids' diets as a communal endeavor" and work to "ensure that parents—*all* parents—have the means necessary to nourish their children" (2021, xxiv).

22 Certainly, some forms of cancer, like lung cancer, are subjected to much the same victim-blaming as diabetes.

23 Richard M. Mizelle Jr. offers an important account of the causes and effects of disproportionate rates of diabetic amputations in communities of color, arguing that amputations offer "a window into the stark realities of diabetes, race, and exclusion in the USA" (2021, 1256).

24 The poem appears to be explicitly in conversation with *Decolonize Your Diet*, a food justice project by Luz Calvo and Catriona Rueda Esquibel that began as a class at Cal State East Bay, where Calvo is a professor of ethnic studies, and evolved into a website and published cookbook (Calvo and Esquibel 2015).

3. HEALING WITHOUT A CURE

1 This means I've made the heartbreaking decision not to examine Machado's memoir *In the Dream House*, a text that shatters me and then puts me back

together again every time I read it. Even though Machado's memoir doesn't quite meet my selection principles for this chapter, I still recommend it to everyone interested in literary representations of domestic abuse—and that likely includes you, if you haven't already read it.

2 I am grateful to Hershini Bhana Young for pushing me to foreground this point. Even while emphasizing that intimate partner violence is not merely an individual health concern, it is worth noting that the health effects of domestic abuse are wide-ranging and well documented. Public health scholar and intimate partner violence expert Tricia Bent-Goodley (2007), for instance, cites an expansive range of studies showing its physical and mental health effects. The list she compiles is astonishing in its breadth: "IPV is connected to higher levels of hypertension, diabetes, pain syndromes, miscarriage, abortion, insomnia, fatigue, urinary tract infections, irritable bowel syndrome, arthritis, chronic disability, migraines, stomach ulcers, HIV/AIDS, and sexually transmitted diseases" (91), as well as to increased "feelings of fearfulness, depression, anxiety, posttraumatic stress disorder (PTSD), suicidal ideation, loss of self-efficacy, and substance abuse" (92).

3 It is important to recognize that *feminicide* refers to the most extreme outcome of heteropatriarchal violence: death. Still, even though most of the texts discussed in this chapter do not depict this most extreme outcome, I find the work of the Latin American and Latina feminist scholars responding to feminicidal violence crucial to my analysis. It is important to note that intimate partner violence often leads to death, with the Centers for Disease Control and Prevention (2021) reporting that one in five of all US homicide victims are killed by an intimate partner and more than half of all US female murder victims are killed by a current or former male intimate partner.

4 According to the biography on Nazario's website, enriquesjourney.com, she is at work on a second book. Given that her first book emerged out of a series of articles for the *Los Angeles Times*—and given the repetition of themes and tropes across these *New York Times* pieces—it seems likely that these articles are part of that new project.

5 Saidiya Hartman's critique of empathy and melodrama figures heavily in Puga's development of the concept of the migrant melodrama, especially in later work with coauthor Víctor M. Espinosa (2020). I will also discuss Hartman's work later in this chapter.

6 Nazario repeats these arguments across multiple editorials and essays, varying the wording slightly each time. For instance, the argument that the United States can accommodate the relatively small number of Central American asylum seekers surfaces at least three times. From an op-ed published in July 2018: "In the first nine months of this fiscal year, 68,560 families and 37,450 unaccompanied children were apprehended at our southern border. That's not a 'flood.' It's one football stadium of people. We can afford

that level of compassion in this country" (2018a). From an op-ed published in October 2018: "This fiscal year, 50,036 unaccompanied migrant children were apprehended coming to the United States. They wouldn't even fill up half a Penn State football stadium. That's refugee dust, as one friend quipped" (2018b). And, finally, from her long-form essay from July 2019: "In the last fiscal year, 97,728 migrants had a credible-fear interview, the first step in the asylum process for people who fear being returned to their own country. Only a small percentage will ultimately be approved. There is no public breakdown on asylum applications by gender, but if even half of those were domestic violence cases, it would be an entirely manageable number of people for one of the richest countries in the world to take in" (2019b).

7   I say that the matter has not been definitively settled in US immigration law because the Sessions ruling that domestic violence be treated as a private brutality rather than political persecution was quickly blocked by a judge and later vacated by Attorney General Merrick Garland (appointed by Trump's successor, Joe Biden). As of this writing, the case has not been tested before a higher court, leaving the asylum cases of abuse survivors vulnerable to the political whims of Garland's successors.

8   Music critic Ann Powers (2014a) refers to Hurray for the Riff Raff as a "collective" rather than a band, a description that might seem counterintuitive since the group's recordings entirely follow Segarra's vision. However, this characterization makes sense when one considers the role of fiddler Yosi Perlstein, who appeared on every Hurray for the Riff Raff album prior to 2017's *The Navigator*. In a (rare) interview with a New Zealand queer website in 2014, Perlstein identifies Segarra as the group's leader, stating that Segarra "started Hurray for the Riff Raff . . . and I joined the band a couple years later" and that "I personally am not very involved on the industry side of things" (*Gay Express* 2014). Meanwhile, in an interview with *OffBeat Magazine* after the release of *The Navigator*, Segarra describes Perlstein's departure as a shift in their own vision for the group:

> Yosi decided he didn't want to tour anymore and wanted to live his life in Tennessee. So that was another really big change for me. It felt like I lost my partner in crime, you know, and this total comfort of having this person who'd been with me for so long. I felt like I'm finally riding solo now. And that's the thing about having a band where you're the songwriter. You gotta let people also live their lives. (A. Johnson 2017)

Thus, although many critics attribute the change in Hurray for the Riff Raff's sound on *The Navigator* to Segarra's reclaiming of their heritage, their comments on Perlstein's departure (and the loss of the fiddle as a crucial element of the group's sound) suggest an interdependency between Segarra and their collaborators that is often overlooked.

9   I have not come across interviews in which Segarra comments on the fact that "Delia's Gone" is specifically about the murder of a Black woman, and

given the fact that Delia's race is not mentioned in the song (whose lyrics are particularly misogynistic and violent), it is possible that Segarra was not aware of the racial dimensions of the song, which is abhorrent for many reasons. For that reason, I don't base my analysis exclusively on Delia's race, but given Segarra's own racial politics, I do find it significant that the murder ballad they specifically call out in the song is one about the death of a Black woman.

10 Segarra scrubs their Instagram each time they release a new album. This is both frustrating and helpful for those seeking to write about them: it definitely makes their Instagram easier to navigate even as it precludes access to older content.

11 The video can be viewed on the online platform YouTube (Hurray for the Riff Raff 2014a).

12 Trayvon Martin, a Black teenager, was shot and killed by a neighborhood watch volunteer in Florida in 2012. The reference to Fulton is further underscored by the fact that Segarra donated proceeds from the video to the Third Wave Fund and the Trayvon Martin Foundation.

13 Kulbaga and Spencer (2019) note that the idea of common sense is frequently invoked to define both violence and consent in sexual encounters, contributing to a "purposeful ambiguity" (3) around both concepts: "We are interested in productively problematizing the idea that consent is plain common sense, especially given the ways in which the rhetoric of 'common sense' can be used to discredit the need for research and policy. As is so often the case when appeals to common sense are used, normative and inaccurate concepts flow in to fill the cracks left by the lack of a clear definition. And normative and inaccurate concepts . . . are part of the problem" (3). In this chapter as a whole, I am suggesting that cultural criticism is one kind of research that can dislodge the prevailing discourse of common sense.

14 Advocates frequently state that the most dangerous time in an abusive relationship is when the victim is leaving. Natasha Trethewey's searing 2020 book *Memorial Drive: A Daughter's Memoir* provides a heart-wrenching literary account of what this danger looks like.

15 Delise Wear and Julie M. Aultman, who have used literature in medical education with the goal of training more "empathetic" doctors, have observed precisely this failure: "As long as the characters exhibit little defiance or disrespect of doctors or mainstream western medicine; as long as they are fairly 'traditional,' particularly regarding sexual orientation; and as long as they exhibit some consistency in making 'good' life choices, students generally are open to engaging with the literature we select. When fictional others fall outside these parameters, students are very apt to resist the text and any discussion of issues related to it" (2005, 1057).

16 One particularly well-known journalistic account of these migrations can be found in Rubén Martínez's *Crossing Over* (2002), which follows the

Chávez family in their back-and-forth migrations from the town of Cherán, Michoacán, located less than an hour's drive from Zacapu.

17 González writes: "In México the homosexual has many names: joto, puto, marica, maricon, margarita, and my favorite, *mariposa*, butterfly, an allusion to the feminine fluttering of eyelashes" (2006, 184). For more on the use of the butterfly as a symbol of Latinx queer masculinity, see Daniel Pérez 2014; on its use as a symbol in migrant rights activism, see S. Wald 2016.

18 The first time I heard Cruz make this statement was at a reading from a draft of the novel in 2013, given at the first Biennial Latina/o Literary Theory and Criticism Conference, organized by Richard Pérez and Belinda Linn Rincón at the John Jay College of Criminal Justice. For a decade now, this labor of love from Pérez and Rincón has provided a generative intellectual environment that has yielded too many insights about Latinx literature to recount, but Cruz's 2013 reading was particularly memorable for me.

19 Although Ana specifically frames her decision as choosing her family over César, the novel suggests that Ana's explanation is something of an oversimplification. Indeed, the relationship between César and Ana is quite complicated. The text suggests in places that César and Ana are natural allies because they are both recipients of Juan's violence, which in the darker-skinned César's case is racialized rather than gendered. In other places, however, there are hints that César might not be completely reliable: he defends Juan to Ana, telling her at one point that Juan "can be an asshole, but he's not a bad guy" (Cruz 2019, 104); during their brief affair, Ana is never entirely certain that César is faithful to her. Although analyzing this relationship is beyond the scope of this project, what is important to underscore is the way Cruz renders César a mostly likable character but also denies him the role of Ana's rescuer. If the overlap of colonial, white supremacist and heteropatriarchal institutions is the root of Ana's oppression, Cruz insists, then replacing her current heteronormative marriage with another will not guarantee her liberation.

4. MENTAL HEALTH AND MIGRANT JUSTICE

1 The administrations that preceded Trump's separated migrant families when a child was deemed to be in danger or the parents were suspected of criminal activity. After Trump rescinded the "zero tolerance" policy, immigration authorities continued separating families in such cases, meaning that the decision to separate was left up to individual officers, with no standards or oversight in place (Thompson 2018).

2 See Dickerson 2020 for a report about families that have not been reunited. See Martin 2021 for a profile of one family experiencing the ongoing effects of the separations.

3 I don't find the distinction between "lawful" and "unlawful" immigration useful, because immigration laws are neither natural nor fixed but politically

determined, but it is worth restating here that Nielsen was *not* "enforcing the law" by implementing zero tolerance; US law permits refugees to present themselves at border checkpoints to request asylum.

4   I discuss critiques of *Enrique's Journey* by Marta Caminero-Santangelo (2012), Monica Hanna (2016), and Ana Elena Puga (2016) in chapter 3.

5   Although Trump's administration is not the only US regime to engage in the systemic abuse of children, his policy does provide one particularly clear example of how this works. Even as women associated with his administration—like Ivanka Trump and Secretary Nielsen—declared the need to protect children from the danger of border crossing, the child separation policy was deliberately designed to inflict psychological torment on migrant families. A *New York Times* investigation conducted years later makes this clear: top officials in Trump's Justice Department, including former attorney general Jeff Sessions and former deputy attorney general Rod J. Rosenstein, were discovered to have insisted on implementing zero tolerance even as US attorneys on the border (including Trump appointees) expressed concerns about child welfare. "We need to take away children," the report quotes Sessions as insisting (Shear, Benner, and Schmidt 2020).

6   Edelman has been rightfully critiqued for the fact that his polemic against "reproductive futurism" fails to account for the whiteness of the sacralized Child; the most influential of these critiques can be found in the work of José Esteban Muñoz (2009). While I find these critiques immensely important, I do think that immigration reform proposals that assert the innocence of child migrants while leaving their parents vulnerable to deportation and detention engage precisely in the kind of political rhetoric that Edelman critiques, treating the Child as "the perpetual horizon of every acknowledged politics" (2004, 3).

7   Although Operation Gatekeeper was implemented nearly two decades ago and was focused on one very specific location along the US-Mexico border, Joseph Nevins (2002) has convincingly shown that it provided the blueprint for the contemporary and ongoing militarization of the border. The work of sociologist Timothy J. Dunn (1996) is also a helpful source for looking at border policy in the years immediately prior to the implementation of Operation Gatekeeper.

8   It is important to note that Bruce's alignment of fugitivity and diaspora with madness is rooted in his engagement with the afterlives of slavery; without comparing slavery to undocumented migration (both distinct forms of racial injustice produced by racial capitalism), I find his language apt in this context.

9   In fact, it was my desire to teach *The Distance between Us* that inspired me to try out a strategy that I now regularly employ when teaching difficult or controversial texts, which is to offer a choice of readings along with extensive content notes *and* ground rules for discussion.

10 The Díaz controversy has often been described as a #MeToo scandal because some of the instances of aggressive behavior included sexual advances; I do not characterize it in this way because not all of the accusations—like that of the queer, disabled Chicano writer Alex Espinoza (2018), which highlights homophobic and ableist bullying—involve sexual misconduct.

11 The Díaz controversy produced dozens of open letters, blog posts, think pieces, Twitter threads, and more, most of which I do not cite here. Gil'Adí's article offers both a helpful bibliography of this writing and an insightful, nuanced analysis of it.

12 As Elda María Román notes, the events of Yunior's life as depicted in Díaz's three books sometimes conflict; she offers a useful way of thinking about these contradictions: "Given Díaz's fondness for science fiction, it is not a stretch to see these . . . stories as exercises in depicting alternate realities" (2017, 108). Following Román, I suggest that it is not a stretch to see Yunior himself as an exercise in imagining alternate realities for Díaz.

13 Although Yunior does not describe sexual abuse as explicitly as Díaz does in "The Silence," he is sexually assaulted during his childhood. The most graphic description takes place in "Ysrael," the first story in *Drown*, which narrates an incident on a public bus when a man pinches his penis through his shorts and smiles; later, when Yunior starts to cry, his older brother calls him a "pussy" (Díaz 1996, 13).

14 Here again Carter (2021) is useful: "Second, I argue that the current over-attention placed on the so-called traumatic 'events of origin' is misguided and that definitions of trauma must be untethered from the 'event(s)' that may initiate it. Focusing solely on the etiologies of trauma risks yielding a hierarchy of 'what counts' as trauma and what events are 'traumatic' enough."

15 Román supports this reading with exquisitely observed textual details, noting that the first story in *Drown* depicts Yunior living in a three-room house in Santo Domingo, whereas *This Is How You Lose Her* concludes with a story that describes his apartment in Cambridge overlooking Harvard.

16 The Salvadoran Civil War, fought between the US-backed military junta government of El Salvador and the Farabundo Martí National Liberation Front (FMLN), began on October 15, 1979, with a military coup, and ended on January 19, 1992, with the signing of the Chapultepec Peace Accords.

17 As I was preparing this chapter for final submission to the press for publication, Zamora published a rigorously detailed memoir of this journey (Zamora 2022), which Karla Cornejo Villavicencio (2022) compares in her *New York Times* review to a reporter's notebook in which "everything is described meticulously so that it can be remembered." Readers of *Solito*, Zamora's memoir, might be surprised by my choice to highlight interview passages in which Zamora claims a sparse or episodic memory, but I argue

that both can be true at once and that the different stylistic choices made by Zamora in his prose and poetry accounts highlight how traumatic memories can be both incomplete and starkly detailed. As Cornejo (2022) insightfully observes, the memoir is both a migration story and "an artist's coming-of-age story" in which Zamora "becomes the narrator of his own life." I wish the publication schedule for this book had allowed more time for me to explore this idea, and eagerly look forward to reading the literary study that does so.

18 Hanna uses the English word *chronicle* to describe this genre rather than the Spanish *crónica*, even though the latter is a widely recognized Latin American literary genre; this choice highlights "the historicity of this writing, the dominance of English language writing among practitioners in the genre, and these writers' formative connections to Anglophone US traditions that intersect with the crónica" (2016, 364). This choice feels right to me for an analysis of Cornejo's work as well, because although readers of Latin American *cronistas* like José Martí, Carlos Monsiváis, or Elena Poniatowska might see her work as reminiscent of theirs, Cornejo herself insistently cites the influence of US-based literary journalists like Charles Bowden (see, for instance, Iberico Lozada 2020). This move, furthermore, recalls my discussion of Amy Moran-Thomas's reframing of the *crónica* genre in chapter 2 of this book.

REMEDIO: THE NAVIGATOR

1 Critics repeatedly note the influence of Bikini Kill on Segarra, who often announces their arrival onstage at shows with the iconic Bikini Kill song "Rebel Girl." Depending on which Hurray for the Riff Raff album is being reviewed, Bikini Kill is sometimes described as a starting point and sometimes as an end point for their sound. Reviewing the bluegrass-influenced *Small Town Heroes*, Stephen M. Deusner (2014) describes Segarra as "a Bronx-born Puerto Rican who gravitated toward Bikini Kill before discovering Woody Guthrie," while Matthew Ismael Ruiz (2017), reviewing *The Navigator*, describes them as "a Nuyorican runaway who grew up obsessed with *West Side Story* before being liberated by Bikini Kill."

2 I use she/her pronouns for Navi throughout this remedio and they/them pronouns for Segarra. Prior to the release of the 2022 album *Life on Earth*, including during the time when they were recording and touring on *The Navigator*, Segarra used she/her pronouns; they have also consistently used she/her pronouns for Navi in interviews. Because I do hold the literary critic's commitment to differentiating character from author, I find using different pronouns for Segarra and for Navi helpful not only as a stylistic device but also as an interpretive device.

3 This happened at a show I attended with my best-friend-forever-for-life, Kaidra L. Mitchell, in Vancouver in June 2017, and the effect was powerful: the Canadian audience (which had already struck me as more polite than

the US audiences with whom I typically attend shows) immediately and shamefacedly complied; for the rest of the show, if *anyone* tried to speak to a companion, someone else would immediately shush them.

4 Regarding the "Hungry Ghost" video, Segarra told *The Fader*: "'Hungry Ghost' captures the beauty of safe and queer DIY venues and parties. . . . With those we lost in Oakland and Orlando in our hearts, this video is a love letter to all the queer people who are putting on intentional events that promote nights of safety, unity and freedom. Keep up the good work" (Mandel 2017). The video for "Pa'lante" is a short film depicting the aftermath of Hurricane Maria, created by Puerto Rican film director Kristian Mercado (Díaz-Hurtado 2018).

5 I use the language of "we" here, aligning myself with those in my family who have abused my sister, although it doesn't quite feel right to do so. *I don't want to believe that I have participated in this.* Every time I read these sentences I try desperately to find another way to phrase this, but it feels even more dishonest to present myself as my sister's sole supporter or even "savior." I feel compelled to acknowledge that as much as I have worked to align myself away from my family's racism and ableism, these ideologies have inevitably shaped me. The language of "we" makes me deeply uncomfortable, but I use it to hold myself accountable.

6 I elaborate the racialized contours of this violence in the introduction to this book.

7 It is worth emphasizing that Metzl's book was published in 2019, before the onset of the COVID-19 pandemic, which likely exacerbated the very trends he highlights.

REFERENCES

Abrajano, Marisa, and Zoltan L. Hajnal. 2015. *White Backlash: Immigration, Race, and American Politics*. Princeton, NJ: Princeton University Press.

Aho, Tanja, Liat Ben-Moshe, and Leon J. Hilton. 2017. "Mad Futures: Affect/Theory/Violence." *American Quarterly* 69, no. 2: 291–302.

Allatson, Paul. 2007. "'My Bones Shine in the Dark': AIDS and the De-scription of Chicano Queer in the Work of Gil Cuadros." *Aztlán: A Journal of Chicano Studies* 32, no. 1: 23–52.

Alvarado, Leticia. 2018. *Abject Performances: Aesthetic Strategies in Latino Cultural Production*. Durham, NC: Duke University Press.

Alvarez, Stephanie. 2006. "¡¿Qué, qué?! Transculturación and Tato Laviera's Spanglish Poetics." *CENTRO Journal* 28, no. 2: 25–47.

Anguiano, Claudia A., and Karma R. Chávez. 2011. "DREAMers' Discourse: Young Latino/a Immigrants and the Naturalization of the American Dream." In *Latina/o Discourse in Vernacular Spaces: Somos de una voz?*, edited by Michelle A. Holling and Bernadette Marie Calafell, 81–99. Lanham, MD: Lexington Books.

Anzaldúa, Gloria. 2002. "now let us shift . . . the path of conocimiento . . . inner work, public acts." In *This Bridge We Call Home: Radical Visions for Transformation*, edited by Gloria E. Anzaldúa and AnaLouise Keating, 540–78. New York: Routledge.

Arenas, Reinaldo. 1992. *Antes que anochezca*. Barcelona: Tusquets.

Avila, Eric. 2004. *Popular Culture in the Age of White Flight: Fear and Fantasy in Suburban Los Angeles*. Berkeley: University of California Press.

Bailey, Moya, and Izetta Autumn Mobley. 2019. "Work in the Intersections: A Black Feminist Disability Framework." *Gender and Society* 33, no. 1: 19–40.

Balaban, Samantha. 2019. "'Just Ask!' Says Sonia Sotomayor. She Knows What It's Like to Feel Different." *NPR*, September 1, 2019. https://www.npr.org/sections /health-shots/2019/09/01/755845325/just-ask-says-sonia-sotomayor-she-knows -what-its-like-to-feel-different.

Banner, Olivia. 2016. "Structural Racism and Practices of Reading in the Medical Humanities." *Literature and Medicine* 34, no. 1: 25–52.

Bansinath, Bindu. 2019. "She Couldn't Find Dominican Women in the Official Archive. So She Started Her Own." *The Cut*, October 31, 2019. https://www.thecut .com/2019/10/angie-cruz-on-her-instagram-archive-dominicanas-nyc.html.

Barrish, Phillip J. 2016. "Health Policy in Dystopia." *Literature and Medicine* 34, no. 1: 106–31.

Baynton, Douglas C. 2016. *Defectives in the Land: Disability and Immigration in the Age of Eugenics*. Chicago: University of Chicago Press.

Bebout, Lee. 2016. *Whiteness on the Border: Mapping the U.S. Racial Imagination in Brown and White*. New York: New York University Press.

Bell, Chris. 2006. "Introducing White Disability Studies: A Modest Proposal." In *The Disability Studies Reader*, edited by Lennard J. Davis, 275–82. New York: Routledge.

Bell, Chris. 2012. "I'm Not the Man I Used to Be: Sex, HIV, and Cultural 'Responsibility.'" In *Sex and Disability*, edited by Robert McRuer and Anna Mollow, 208–28. Durham, NC: Duke University Press.

Beltrán, Cristina. 2010. *The Trouble with Unity: Latino Politics and the Creation of Identity*. Oxford: Oxford University Press.

Benner, Katie, and Caitlin Dickerson. 2018. "Sessions Says Domestic and Gang Violence Are Not Grounds for Asylum." *New York Times*, June 11, 2018. https:// www.nytimes.com/2018/06/11/us/politics/sessions-domestic-violence-asylum .html.

Bent-Goodley, Tricia B. 2007. "Health Disparities and Violence against Women: Why and How Cultural and Societal Influences Matter." *Trauma, Violence and Abuse* 8, no. 2: 90–104.

Berlant, Lauren. 2007. "Slow Death (Sovereignty, Obesity, Lateral Agency)." *Critical Inquiry* 33, no. 4: 754–80.

Berlant, Lauren. 2011. *Cruel Optimism*. Durham, NC: Duke University Press.

Berne, Patty. 2015. "Disability Justice—a Working Draft by Patty Berne." *Sins Invalid*, June 9, 2015. https://www.sinsinvalid.org/blog/disability-justice-a -working-draft-by-patty-berne.

Biltekoff, Charlotte. 2013. *Eating Right in America: The Cultural Politics of Food and Health*. Durham, NC: Duke University Press.

Blitzer, Jonathan. 2017. "An Immigrant Who Crossed the Border as a Child Retraces His Journey, in Poems." *New Yorker*, September 19, 2017. https://www

.newyorker.com/books/page-turner/an-immigrant-who-crossed-the-border-as
-a-child-retraces-his-journey-in-poems.

Bolton, Sony Coráñez. 2023. *Crip Colony: Mestizaje, US Imperialism, and the Queer Politics of Disability in the Philippines*. Durham, NC: Duke University Press.

Bonilla-Silva, Eduardo. 2014. *Racism without Racists: Color-Blind Racism and the Persistence of Racial Inequality in America*. 4th ed. Lanham, MD: Rowman and Littlefield.

Bost, Suzanne. 2010. *Encarnación: Illness and Body Politics in Chicana Feminist Literature*. New York: Fordham University Press.

Bost, Suzanne. 2015. "Messy Archives and Materials That Matter: Making Knowledge with the Gloria Evangelina Anzaldúa Papers." *PMLA* 130, no. 3: 615–30.

Briggs, Laura. 2003. *Reproducing Empire: Race, Sex, Science, and U.S. Imperialism in Puerto Rico*. Berkeley: University of California Press.

Briggs, Laura. 2017. *How All Politics Became Reproductive Politics: From Welfare Reform to Foreclosure to Trump*. Berkeley: University of California Press.

Bruce, La Marr Jurelle. 2021. *How to Go Mad without Losing Your Mind: Madness and Black Radical Creativity*. Durham, NC: Duke University Press.

Cabreja, Karina Maria. 2018. "The Reckoning: What Junot Díaz Teaches Us about Internalized Misogyny." *The Root*, May 5, 2018. https://www.theroot.com/the -reckoning-what-junot-diaz-teaches-us-about-interna-1825796965.

Cacho, Lisa Marie. 2012. *Social Death: Racialized Rightlessness and the Criminalization of the Unprotected*. New York: New York University Press.

Calvo, Luz, and Catriona Rueda Esquibel. 2015. *Decolonize Your Diet: Plant-Based Mexican-American Recipes for Health and Healing*. Vancouver, BC: Arsenal Pulp.

Caminero-Santangelo, Marta. 2012. "Narrating the Non-nation: Literary Journalism and 'Illegal' Border Crossings." *Arizona Quarterly* 68, no. 3: 157–76.

Caminero-Santangelo, Marta. 2016. *Documenting the Undocumented: Latino/a Narratives and Social Justice in the Era of Operation Gatekeeper*. Gainesville: University Press of Florida.

Campo, Rafael. 1996. *What the Body Told*. Durham, NC: Duke University Press.

Campo, Rafael. 1998. *The Desire to Heal: A Doctor's Education in Empathy, Identity, and Poetry*. New York: Norton.

Campo, Rafael. 2013a. *Alternative Medicine*. Durham, NC: Duke University Press.

Campo, Rafael. 2013b. "Wednesday HIV Clinic." *Journal of Medical Humanities* 34, no. 2: 285–87.

Campo, Rafael. 2018. *Comfort Measures Only: New and Selected Poems, 1994–2016*. Durham, NC: Duke University Press.

Cancryn, Adam, and Laura Barrón-López. 2020. "Azar Faulted Workers' 'Home and Social' Conditions for Meatpacking Outbreaks." *Politico*, May 7, 2020. https://www .politico.com/news/2020/05/07/azar-coronavirus-meatpacking-workers-241915.

Capelouto, J. D. 2019. "Ban the Dollar Store? Local Communities Halt New Discount Shops." *Atlanta Journal-Constitution*, December 17, 2019. https://www .ajc.com/news/local/ban-the-dollar-store-stonecrest-dekalb-halt-new-ones /pQNHyOIgAJmkCGjuhp22QI/.

Capps, Randy, Michael Fix, and Jie Zong. 2016. *A Profile of U.S. Children with Unauthorized Immigrant Parents*. Washington, DC: Migration Policy Institute. https://www.migrationpolicy.org/sites/default/files/publications /ChildrenofUnauthorized-FactSheet-FINAL.pdf.

Carter, Angela M. 2021. "When Silence Said Everything: Reconceptualizing Trauma through Critical Disability Studies." *Lateral* 10, no. 1. https://csalateral .org/section/cripistemologies-of-crisis/when-silence-said-everything -reconceptualizing-trauma-through-critical-disability-studies-carter/.

Castañeda, Heide, Seth M. Holmes, Daniel S. Madrigal, Maria-Elena DeTrinidad Young, Naomi Beyeler, and James Quesada. 2015. "Immigration as a Social Determinant of Health." *Annual Review of Public Health* 36:375–92.

Center for HIV Law and Policy. 2022. "HIV Criminalization in the United States: A Sourcebook on State and Federal HIV Criminal Law and Practice." Updated February 2022. https://www.hivlawandpolicy.org/sourcebook.

Centers for Disease Control and Prevention. 2021. "Preventing Intimate Partner Violence." November 2, 2021. https://www.cdc.gov/violenceprevention /intimatepartnerviolence/fastfact.html.

Chandler, Adam. 2015. "Why the Fast-Food Ban Failed in South L.A." *Atlantic*, March 24, 2015. https://www.theatlantic.com/health/archive/2015/03/why-the -fast-food-ban-failed-in-south-la/388475/.

Charon, Rita. 2006. *Narrative Medicine: Honoring the Stories of Illness*. Oxford: Oxford University Press.

Chasman, Deborah, and Joshua Cohen. 2018. "A Letter from Deborah Chasman and Joshua Cohen." *Boston Review*, June 5, 2018. http://bostonreview.net/editors -note/boston-review-letter-deborah-chasman-and-joshua-cohen.

Chávez, Karma R. 2021. *The Borders of AIDS: Race, Quarantine, and Resistance*. Seattle: University of Washington Press.

Cházaro, Angélica, and Jennifer Casey. 2006. "Getting Away with Murder: Guatemala's Failure to Protect Women and Rodi Alvarado's Quest for Safety." *Hastings Women's Law Journal* 17, no. 2: 141–86.

Chen, Ching-In, Jai Dulani, and Leah Lakshmi Piepzna-Samarasinha, eds. 2016. *The Revolution Starts at Home: Confronting Intimate Violence within Activist Communities*. 2nd ed. Chico, CA: AK Press.

Cheng, Jih-Fei, Alexandra Juhasz, and Nishant Shahani. 2020. Introduction to *AIDS and the Distribution of Crises*, 1–28. Durham, NC: Duke University Press.

Cisneros, Sandra. (1984) 1991. *The House on Mango Street*. New York: Vintage Contemporaries.

Cisneros, Sandra. 1992. *Woman Hollering Creek and Other Stories*. New York: Vintage.

Clare, Eli. 2017. *Brilliant Imperfection: Grappling with Cure*. Durham, NC: Duke University Press.

Combahee River Collective. (1983) 2000. "The Combahee River Collective Statement." In *Home Girls: A Black Feminist Anthology*, edited by Barbara Smith, 264–74. New Brunswick, NJ: Rutgers University Press.

Cornejo Villavicencio, Karla. 2020. *The Undocumented Americans*. New York: One World.

Cornejo Villavicencio, Karla. 2021. "In Utopia, I Never Have to Write about Immigration Again." *Nation*, July 26/August 2, 2021. https://www.thenation.com/article/society/immigration-art-borders/.

Cornejo Villavicencio, Karla. 2022. "The Harrowing Migration Story of One 9-Year-Old Child." *New York Times*, September 8, 2022. https://www.nytimes.com/2022/09/08/books/review/solito-javier-zamora.html.

Cortez, Jaime. 2004. *Sexile/Sexilio*. Los Angeles: Institute for Gay Men's Health.

Cowing, Jess L. 2020. "Occupied Land Is an Access Issue: Interventions in Feminist Disability Studies and Narratives of Indigenous Activism." *Journal of Feminist Scholarship*, no. 17, 9–25.

Crawford, Lucas. 2017. "Slender Trouble: From Berlant's Cruel Figuring of Figure to Sedgwick's Fat Presence." GLQ 23, no. 4: 447–72.

Crawford, Robert. 1980. "Healthism and the Medicalization of Everyday Life." *International Journal of Health Services* 10, no. 3: 365–88.

Cruz, Angie. 2019. *Dominicana*. New York: Flatiron Books.

Cruz, Angie, and Nelly Rosario. 2007. "Angie Cruz in Conversation with Nelly Rosario." *Callaloo: A Journal of African Diaspora Arts and Letters* 30, no. 3: 743–53.

Cuadros, Gil. 1994. *City of God*. San Francisco: City Lights Books.

Cutler, John Alba. 2015. *Ends of Assimilation: The Formation of Chicano Literature*. Oxford: Oxford University Press.

Cvetkovich, Ann. 2003. *An Archive of Feelings: Trauma, Sexuality, and Lesbian Public Cultures*. Durham, NC: Duke University Press.

Cvetkovich, Ann. 2012. *Depression: A Public Feeling*. Durham, NC: Duke University Press.

Dalleo, Raphael, and Elena Machado Sáez. 2007. *The Latino/a Canon and the Emergence of Post-Sixties Literature*. New York: Palgrave Macmillan.

Daniels, Caitlin. 2016. "Economic Constraints on Taste Formation and the True Cost of Healthy Eating." *Social Science and Medicine* 148:34–41.

Danticat, Edwidge. 1995. *Breath, Eyes, Memory*. New York: Vintage.

Davis, Lennard. 2002. *Bending over Backwards: Disability, Dismodernism, and Other Difficult Positions*. New York: New York University Press.

Dean, Tim. 2009. *Unlimited Intimacy: Reflections on the Subculture of Barebacking*. Chicago: University of Chicago Press.

Decena, Carlos Ulises. 2008. "Profiles, Compulsory Disclosure, and Ethical Sexual Citizenship in the Contemporary USA." *Sexualities* 11, no. 4: 397–413.

deOnís, Catalina (Kathleen). 2017. "What's in an 'X'? An Exchange about the Politics of 'Latinx.'" *Chiricú Journal* 1, no. 2: 78–91.

Deusner, Stephen M. 2014. "*Small Town Heroes*: Hurray for the Riff Raff." *Pitchfork*, February 18, 2014. https://pitchfork.com/reviews/albums/19031-hurray-for-the-riff-raff-small-town-heroes/.

Díaz, Junot. 1996. *Drown*. New York: Riverhead.

Díaz, Junot. 2007. *The Brief Wondrous Life of Oscar Wao*. New York: Riverhead.

Díaz, Junot. 2012. *This Is How You Lose Her*. New York: Riverhead.

Díaz, Junot. 2018. "The Silence: The Legacy of Childhood Trauma." *New Yorker*, April 9, 2018. https://www.newyorker.com/magazine/2018/04/16/the-silence -the-legacy-of-childhood-trauma.

Díaz-Hurtado, Jessica. 2018. "A Recovering Puerto Rico Stars in Hurray for the Riff Raff's 'Pa'lante' Video." *NPR Alt.Latino*, May 21, 2018. https://www.npr.org /sections/altlatino/2018/05/21/613052812/a-recovering-puerto-rico-stars-in -hurray-for-the-riff-raffs-palante-video.

Dickerson, Caitlin. 2019. "The Youngest Child Separated from His Family at the Border Was 4 Months Old." *New York Times*, June 16, 2019. https://www .nytimes.com/2019/06/16/us/baby-constantine-romania-migrants.html.

Dickerson, Caitlin. 2020. "Parents of 545 Children Separated at the Border Cannot Be Found." *New York Times*, October 21, 2020. https://www.nytimes.com/2020 /10/21/us/migrant-children-separated.html.

Diedrich, Lisa. 2005. "AIDS and Its Treatments: Two Doctors' Narratives of Heal-ing, Desire, and Belonging." *Journal of Medical Humanities* 26, no. 4: 237–57.

Doucleff, Michaeleen. 2016. "Researchers Clear 'Patient Zero' from AIDS Origin Story." *NPR*, October 26, 2016. https://www.npr.org/sections/health-shots/2016 /10/26/498876985/mystery-solved-how-hiv-came-to-the-u-s.

Dunn, Timothy J. 1996. *The Militarization of the U.S.-Mexico Border, 1978–1992: Low-Intensity Conflict Doctrine Comes Home.* Austin: University of Texas Press.

Edelman, Lee. 2004. *No Future: Queer Theory and the Death Drive.* Durham, NC: Duke University Press.

Eils, Colleen Gleeson. 2017. "Narrating Privacy: Evading Ethnographic Surveillance in Fiction by Sherman Alexie, Rigoberto González, and Nam Le." *MELUS* 42, no. 2: 30–52.

Ellis, Amanda. 2017. "Border Arte as Medicine: Healing beyond the Confines of Our Skin." *Chicana/Latina Studies* 17, no. 1: 30–59.

Ellis, Amanda. 2021. *Letras y Limpias: Decolonial Medicine and Holistic Healing in Mexican American Literature.* Tucson: University of Arizona Press.

Ensler, Eve. 1998. *The Vagina Monologues.* New York: Villard.

Epstein, Reid J. 2014. "NCLR Head: Obama 'Deporter-in-Chief.'" *Politico*, March 4, 2014. https://www.politico.com/story/2014/03/national-council-of-la-raza-janet -murguia-barack-obama-deporter-in-chief-immigration-104217.

Erevelles, Nirmala. 2011. *Disability and Difference in Global Contexts: Enabling a Transformative Body Politic.* New York: Palgrave Macmillan.

Erman, Sam. 2019. *Almost Citizens: Puerto Rico, the U.S. Constitution, and Empire.* Cambridge: Cambridge University Press.

Espinoza, Alex. 2018. Twitter post. May 8, 2018. https://twitter.com/alex_esp/status /993726353642946560.

Facher, Lev. 2017. "Two Months Ago, This Doctor Was Delivering Babies. Now He's at the Nexus of the Obamacare Fight." *STAT*, March 3, 2017. https://www .statnews.com/2017/03/03/roger-marshall-kansas-obamacare/.

Farber, Jim. 2017. "Hurray for the Riff Raff's Alynda Segarra Finds Herself in a Concept Album." *New York Times*, March 8, 2017. https://www.nytimes.com /2017/03/08/arts/music/hurray-for-the-riff-traff-the-navigator-interview.html.

Fensterstock, Alison. 2014. "Behind the Scenes with Katey Red at a Shoot for New Hurray for the Riff Raff Video." *Times-Picayune* (New Orleans), October 9, 2014. https://www.nola.com/entertainment_life/music/article_fe7792f9-6462 -52a1-93e8-9df2c718b0a8.html.

Ferguson, Roderick A. 2004. *Aberrations in Black: Toward a Queer of Color Critique.* Minneapolis: University of Minnesota Press.

Fernández, Johanna. 2020. *The Young Lords: A Radical History.* Chapel Hill: University of North Carolina Press.

Fielding-Singh, Priya. 2017. "A Taste of Inequality: Food's Symbolic Value across the Socioeconomic Spectrum." *Sociological Science* 4:424–48.

Fielding-Singh, Priya. 2021. *How the Other Half Eats: The Untold Story of Food and Inequality in America.* New York: Little, Brown Spark.

Figueroa-Vásquez, Yomaira C. 2020. *Decolonizing Diasporas: Radical Mappings of Afro-Atlantic Literature.* Evanston, IL: Northwestern University Press.

Fink, Sheri. 2018. "Puerto Rico's Hurricane Maria Death Toll Could Exceed 4,000, New Study Estimates." *New York Times*, May 29, 2018.

Flood, Alison. 2018. "Junot Díaz Welcomed Back by Pulitzer Prize after Review into Sexual Misconduct Claims." *Guardian*, November 19, 2018. https://www .theguardian.com/books/2018/nov/19/junot-diaz-welcomed-back-by-pulitzer -prize-after-review-into-sexual-misconduct-claims.

Freeman, Gregory. 2003. "In Search of Death." *Rolling Stone*, February 6, 2003, 44–48.

Fregoso, Rosa-Linda. 2006. "'We Want Them Alive!': The Politics and Culture of Human Rights." *Social Identities* 12, no. 2: 109–38.

Fregoso, Rosa-Linda, and Cynthia Bejarano. 2010. "Introduction: A Cartography of Violence in the Américas." In *Terrorizing Women: Feminicide in the Américas*, edited by Rosa-Linda Fregoso and Cynthia Bejarano, 1–42. Durham, NC: Duke University Press.

Frye, Lezlie. 2016. *Birthing Disability, Reproducing Race: Uneasy Intersections in Post–Civil Rights Politics of U.S. Citizenship.* PhD diss., New York University. ProQuest Number 10191910.

García, Patricia M. 2017. "The 'I' before the Border: An Interview with Reyna Grande." *Symbolism* 17:185–98.

Garcia-Ditta, Alexa. 2015. "Daughter: Mom, Arrested at Gynecology Office, 'Doesn't Deserve What's Going On.'" *Texas Observer*, September 16, 2015. https://www.texasobserver.org/daughter-speaks-out-against-moms-arrest-at -houston-clinic/.

García-Peña, Lorgia. 2016. *The Borders of Dominicanidad: Race, Nation, and Archives of Contradiction.* Durham, NC: Duke University Press.

Garden, Rebecca. 2013. "Distance Learning: Empathy and Culture in Junot Díaz's 'Wildwood.'" *Journal of Medical Humanities* 34, no. 4: 439–50.

Gay, Roxane. 2017. *Hunger: A Memoir of (My) Body.* New York: Harper.

Gay Express. 2014. "Exclusive Interview with Hurray for the Riff Raff's Yosi Perlstein." November 17, 2014. https://gayexpress.co.nz/2014/11/exclusive-interview -hurray-riff-raffs-yosi-perlstien/.

Gil'Adí, Maia. 2020. "'I Think about You, X—': Re-reading Junot Díaz after 'The Silence.'" *Latino Studies* 18, no. 4: 507–30.

Gilmore, Leigh. 2017. *Tainted Witness: Why We Doubt What Women Say about Their Lives*. New York: Columbia University Press.

Gilmore, Ruth Wilson. 2007. *Golden Gulag: Prisons, Surplus, Crisis, and Opposition in Globalizing California*. Berkeley: University of California Press.

González, David. 2010. "Poet Spans Two Worlds, but Has a Home in Neither." *New York Times*, February 12, 2010. https://www.nytimes.com/2010/02/13/nyregion/13poet.html.

González, David. 2013. "Tato Laviera, 63, Poet of Nuyorican School." *New York Times*, November 5, 2013. https://www.nytimes.com/2013/11/06/arts/tato-laviera-nuyorican-poet-dies-at-63.html.

González, Octavio R. 2010. "Tracking the Bugchaser: Giving the Gift of HIV/AIDS." *Cultural Critique*, no. 75 (Spring): 82–113.

González, Rigoberto. 2003. *Crossing Vines*. Norman: University of Oklahoma Press.

González, Rigoberto. 2006. *Butterfly Boy: Memories of a Chicano Mariposa*. Madison: University of Wisconsin Press.

Gordon, Colin. 2003. *Dead on Arrival: The Politics of Health Care in Twentieth-Century America*. Princeton, NJ: Princeton University Press.

Gordon, Colin. 2013. "The Irony and Limits of the Affordable Care Act." *Dissent Magazine* (blog), October 15, 2013. https://www.dissentmagazine.org/online_articles/the-irony-and-limits-of-the-affordable-care-act.

Gordon, Colin. 2018. "Healthy Signs." *Dissent Magazine* (blog), December 19, 2018. https://www.dissentmagazine.org/blog/assessing-affordable-care-act.

Gould, Deborah B. 2009. *Moving Politics: Emotion and ACT UP's Fight against AIDS*. Chicago: University of Chicago Press.

Grande, Reyna. 2006. *Across a Hundred Mountains*. New York: Atria Books.

Grande, Reyna. 2009. *Dancing with Butterflies*. New York: Washington Square.

Grande, Reyna. 2012. *The Distance between Us*. New York: Washington Square.

Grande, Reyna. 2016. *The Distance between Us*. Young Readers Edition. New York: Aladdin.

Grande, Reyna. 2018. "The Impossible Choice My Father Had to Make." *New York Times*, August 11, 2018. https://www.nytimes.com/2018/08/11/opinion/sunday/the-impossible-choice-my-father-had-to-make.html.

Grande, Reyna. 2019. *A Dream Called Home*. New York: Washington Square.

Grise, Virginia. 2017. *Your Healing Is Killing Me*. Pittsburgh, PA: Plays Inverse.

Grise, Virginia, and Irma Mayorga. 2014. *The Panza Monologues*. 2nd ed. Austin: University of Texas Press.

Guthman, Julie. 2011. *Weighing In: Obesity, Food Justice, and the Limits of Capitalism*. Berkeley: University of California Press.

Gutiérrez, Elena R. 2008. *Fertile Matters: The Politics of Mexican-Origin Women's Reproduction*. Austin: University of Texas Press.

Guzmán, Joshua Javier. Forthcoming. *Dissatisfactions: Queer Chicano Style Politics*. New York: New York University Press.

Hall, Kim Q. 2005. "Queerness, Disability, and *The Vagina Monologues*." *Hypatia: A Journal of Feminist Philosophy* 20, no. 1: 99–119.

Hanna, Monica. 2016. "Chronicling Contemporary Latinidad." *American Literature* 88, no. 2: 361–89.

Hartman, Saidiya. 1997. *Scenes of Subjection: Terror, Slavery, and Self-Making in Nineteenth-Century America*. New York: Oxford University Press.

Hartman, Saidiya. 2008. "Venus in Two Acts." *Small Axe*, no. 26, 1–14.

Hatch, Anthony Ryan. 2016. *Blood Sugar: Racial Pharmacology and Food Justice in Black America*. Minneapolis: University of Minnesota Press.

Hebert, Patrick "Pato." 2004. Foreword to *Sexile/Sexilio*, iii–iv. Los Angeles: Institute for Gay Men's Health.

Hennessy-Fiske, Molly. 2020. "Coronavirus Has Torn Texas' Tightknit Rio Grande Valley Apart: 'We're in Hell Right Now.'" *Los Angeles Times*, July 21, 2020. https://www.latimes.com/world-nation/story/2020-07-21/in-texas-rio-grande-valley-familiarity-has-bred-coronavirus.

Hernandez, Kelly Lytle. 2010. *Migra! A History of the U.S. Border Patrol*. Berkeley: University of California Press.

Hey-Colón, Rebeca L. 2022. "Chronic Illness and Transformation in Gloria Anzaldúa's 'Puddles.'" *Aztlán: A Journal of Chicano Studies* 47, no. 1: 15–42.

Holmes, Seth M. 2013. *Fresh Fruit, Broken Bodies: Migrant Farmworkers in the United States*. Berkeley: University of California Press.

Hooper, Molly K. 2009. "'You Lie': Rep. Wilson Apologizes for Yell." *Hill*, September 10, 2009.

Human Impact Partners. 2018. "The Effects of Forced Family Separation in the Rio Grande Valley: A Family Unity, Family Health Research Update." Human Impact Partners, October 2018. https://familyunityfamilyhealth.org/wp-content/uploads/2018/10/HIP-LUPE_FUFH2018-RGV-FullReport.pdf.

Hurray for the Riff Raff. 2013. *My Dearest Darkest Neighbor*. Mod Mobilian Records.

Hurray for the Riff Raff. 2014a. "The Body Electric (Official Video)." *YouTube*, December 11, 2014. https://www.youtube.com/watch?v=_KvXteZkByE.

Hurray for the Riff Raff. 2014b. *Small Town Heroes*. ATO Records.

Hurray for the Riff Raff. 2017. *The Navigator*. ATO Records.

Hurray for the Riff Raff. 2022. *Life on Earth*. Nonesuch Records.

Iberico Lozada, Lucas. 2020. "Karla Cornejo Villavicencio: DREAMer Memoirs Have Their Purpose. But That's Not What I Set Out to Write." *Guernica*, June 10, 2020. https://www.guernicamag.com/karla-cornejo-villavicencio-dreamer-memoirs-have-their-purpose-but-thats-not-what-i-set-out-to-write/.

Inda, Jonathan Xavier. 2020. "Fatal Prescriptions: Immigration Detention, Mismedication, and the Necropolitics of Uncare." *Death Studies* 44, no. 11: 699–708.

Ingraham, Christopher. 2017. "If Jason Chaffetz Wants to Compare Health Care to iPhones, Let's Do It the Right Way." *Washington Post*, March 7, 2017. https://www.washingtonpost.com/news/wonk/wp/2017/03/07/if-jason-chaffetz-wants-to-compare-healthcare-to-iphones-lets-do-it-the-right-way/.

Iwai, Yoshiko, Zahra H. Khan, and Sayantani DasGupta. 2020. "Abolition Medicine." *The Lancet* 396, no. 10245: 158–59.

James, Jennifer C., and Cynthia Wu. 2006. "Editors' Introduction: Race, Ethnicity, Disability, and Literature: Intersections and Interventions." *MELUS* 31, no. 3: 3–13.

Johnson, Alex. 2017. "Backtalk: Alynda Lee Segarra (of Hurray for the Riff Raff)." *OffBeat Magazine*, March 29, 2017. https://www.offbeat.com/articles/backtalk -alynda-lee-segarra-hurray-riff-raff/.

Johnson, Carolyn Y. 2017. "Trump's Pick to Lower Drug Prices Is a Former Pharma Executive Who Raised Them." *Washington Post*, November 13, 2017. https:// www.washingtonpost.com/news/wonk/wp/2017/11/13/trumps-pick-to-lower -drug-prices-is-a-former-pharma-executive-who-raised-them/.

Kafer, Alison. 2013. *Feminist, Queer, Crip.* Bloomington: Indiana University Press.

Kafer, Alison. 2016. "Un/Safe Disclosures: Scenes of Disability and Trauma." *Journal of Literary and Cultural Disability Studies* 10, no. 1: 1–20.

Kafer, Alison, and Eunjung Kim. 2017. "Disability and the Edges of Intersectionality." In *The Cambridge Companion to Literature and Disability*, edited by Clare Barker and Stuart Murray, 123–38. Cambridge: Cambridge University Press.

Kang, Nancy. 2014. "*Butterfly Boy: Memoirs of a Chicano Mariposa* by Rigoberto González (review)." *Callaloo: A Journal of African Diaspora Arts and Letters* 37, no. 3: 750–53.

Kaplan, Ilana. 2017. "Alynda Segarra on Navigating Being Puerto Rican, Queer, and Bronx-Bred." *Nylon*, April 10, 2017. https://www.nylon.com/articles/alynda -segarra-hurray-for-the-riff-raff-interview.

Kates, Graham. 2018. "Migrant Children at the Border—the Facts." *CBS News*, June 20, 2018. https://www.cbsnews.com/news/migrant-children-at-the-border -by-the-numbers/.

Kenney, Julia. 2021. "Peloton's Robin Arzon—'Be Ready for Your Finish Line.'" *DiaTribeLearn*, December 13, 2021. https://diatribe.org/peloton-robin-arzon-be -ready-your-finish-line.

Kim, Eunjung. 2017. *Curative Violence: Rehabilitating Disability, Gender, and Sexuality in Modern Korea.* Durham, NC: Duke University Press.

Kim, Jina B. 2017. "Toward a Crip-of-Color Critique: Thinking with Minich's 'Enabling Whom?'" *Lateral* 6, no. 1. https://csalateral.org/issue/6–1/forum-alt -humanities-critical-disability-studies-crip-of-color-critique-kim/.

Kim, Jina B. 2019. "Love in the Time of Sickness: On Disability, Race, and Intimate Partner Violence." *Asian American Literary Review* 10, no. 2: 191–202.

Kim, Jina B. 2020. "Disability in an Age of Fascism." *American Quarterly* 72, no. 1: 265–76.

Kim, Jina B. 2021. "Cripping the Welfare Queen: The Radical Potential of Disability Politics." *Social Text* 39, no. 3: 79–101.

King, Tiffany Lethabo. 2019. *The Black Shoals: Offshore Formations of Black and Native Studies.* Durham, NC: Duke University Press.

Kirkland, Anna. 2010. "Conclusion: What Next?" In *Against Health: How Health Became the New Morality*, edited by Jonathan M. Metzl and Anna Kirkland, 195–203. New York: New York University Press.

Kirkland, Anna. 2011. "The Environmental Account of Obesity: A Case for Feminist Skepticism." *Signs: Journal of Women in Culture and Society* 36, no. 2: 463–85.

Kirkland, Anna. 2014. "What Is Wellness Now?" *Journal of Health Politics, Policy and Law* 39, no. 5: 957–70.

Klein, Betsy. 2018. "Ivanka Trump: Family Separations Issue 'Was a Low Point.'" *CNN*, August 2, 2018. https://www.cnn.com/2018/08/02/politics/ivanka-trump -immigration-family-separation/index.html.

Kopan, Tal. 2018. "DHS: 2,000 Children Separated from Parents at Border." *CNN*, June 16, 2018. https://www.cnn.com/2018/06/15/politics/dhs-family-separation -numbers/index.html.

Kraut, Alan M. 1994. *Silent Travelers: Germs, Genes, and the "Immigrant Menace."* Baltimore: Johns Hopkins University Press.

Kulbaga, Theresa A., and Leland G. Spencer. 2017. "Fitness and the Feminist First Lady: Gender, Race, and Body in Michelle Obama's *Let's Move!* Campaign." *Women and Language* 40, no. 1: 36–50.

Kulbaga, Theresa A., and Leland G. Spencer. 2019. *Campuses of Consent: Sexual and Social Justice in Higher Education.* Amherst: University of Massachusetts Press.

Lagarde y de los Ríos, Marcela. 2010. "Preface: Feminist Keys for Understanding Feminicide: Theoretical, Political, and Legal Construction." In *Terrorizing Women: Feminicide in the Américas*, edited by Rosa-Linda Fregoso and Cynthia Bejarano, xi–xxv. Durham, NC: Duke University Press.

Laviera, Tato. 2008. *Mixturao and Other Poems.* Houston, TX: Arte Público.

Laviera, Tato. 2014. *Bendición: The Complete Poetry of Tato Laviera.* Houston, TX: Arte Público.

Laviera, Tato, and Stephanie Alvarez. 2014. "Tato in His Own Words: A Collaborative Testimonio." In *The AmeRícan Poet: Essays on the Work of Tato Laviera*, edited by Stephanie A. Alvarez and William Luis, 288–324. New York: CUNY Hunter College Center for Puerto Rican Studies.

Lee, James Kyung-Jin. 2021. *Pedagogies of Woundedness: Illness, Memoir, and the Ends of the Model Minority.* Philadelphia: Temple University Press.

Leonhardt, David. 2016. "A Month without Sugar." *New York Times*, December 30, 2016. https://www.nytimes.com/2016/12/30/opinion/a-month-without-sugar.html.

Leonhardt, David. 2018. "Big Sugar versus Your Body." *New York Times*, March 11, 2018. https://www.nytimes.com/2018/03/11/opinion/sugar-industry-health .html.

Levins Morales, Aurora, and Rosario Morales. 1986. *Getting Home Alive.* Ithaca, NY: Firebrand.

Lew-Williams, Beth. 2018. *The Chinese Must Go: Violence, Exclusion, and the Making of the Alien in America.* Cambridge, MA: Harvard University Press.

Lima, Lázaro. 2007. *The Latino Body: Crisis Identities in American Literary and Cultural Memory.* New York: New York University Press.

Lima, Lázaro. 2019. *Being Brown: Sonia Sotomayor and the Latino Question.* Berkeley: University of California Press.

Lira, Natalie. 2021. *Laboratory of Deficiency: Sterilization and Confinement in California, 1900–1950s*. Berkeley: University of California Press.

Lomas, Laura. 2014a. "Migration and Decolonial Politics in Two Afro-Latino Poets: 'Pachín' Marín and 'Tato' Laviera." *Review: Literature and Art of the Americas* 47, no. 2: 155–63.

Lomas, Laura. 2014b. "'This Is a Warning, My Beloved America': Tato Laviera and the Birth of a New American Poetic Language." In *Bendición: The Complete Poetry of Tato Laviera*, xv–xxviii. Houston, TX: Arte Público.

Loofbourow, Lili. 2018. "Junot Díaz and the Problem of the Male Self-Pardon." *Slate*, June 24, 2018. https://slate.com/culture/2018/06/junot-diaz-allegations -and-the-male-self-pardon.html.

López, Edrik. 2014. "Espanglish: Laviera's el nideaquínideallá Language in Fourteen Movements." In *The AmeRícan Poet: Essays on the Work of Tato Laviera*, edited by Stephanie A. Alvarez and William Luis, 46–62. New York: CUNY Hunter College Center for Puerto Rican Studies.

López, Marissa K. 2019. *Racial Immanence: Chicanx Bodies beyond Representation*. New York: New York University Press.

Lorde, Audre. (1980) 1997. *The Cancer Journals*. Special ed. San Francisco: Aunt Lute Books.

Love, Heather. 2007. *Feeling Backward: Loss and the Politics of Queer History*. Cambridge, MA: Harvard University Press.

Love, Heather. 2012. "What Does Lauren Berlant Teach Us about X?" *Communication and Critical/Cultural Studies* 9, no. 4: 320–36.

Luis, William. 2014. "Introduction: The Life and Rebirths of Tato Laviera." In *The AmeRícan Poet: Essays on the Work of Tato Laviera*, edited by Stephanie A. Alvarez and William Luis, xv–iv. New York: CUNY Hunter College Center for Puerto Rican Studies.

Luna, Caleb. 2016. "Settler Colonialism, Fat Embodiment, and the Biopolitics of Desire." National Women's Studies Association Annual Meeting, Palais des Congrès, Montreal, Session 502, November 13, 2016.

Mac, Ryan, Benjamin Mullin, Kate Conger, and Mike Isaac. 2022. "A Verifiable Mess: Twitter Users Create Havoc by Impersonating Brands." *New York Times*, November 11, 2022. https://www.nytimes.com/2022/11/11/technology/twitter -blue-fake-accounts.html.

Machado, Carmen Maria. 2019. *In the Dream House*. Minneapolis: Graywolf.

Maloney, Jennifer, and Saabira Chaudhuri. 2017. "Against All Odds, the U.S. Tobacco Industry Is Rolling in Money." *Wall Street Journal*, April 23, 2017. https:// www.wsj.com/articles/u-s-tobacco-industry-rebounds-from-its-near-death -experience-1492968698.

Mandavilli, Apoorva. 2019. "H.I.V. Is Reported Cured in a Second Patient, a Milestone in the Global AIDS Epidemic." *New York Times*, March 4, 2019. https:// www.nytimes.com/2019/03/04/health/aids-cure-london-patient.html.

Mandavilli, Apoorva. 2020. "The 'London Patient,' Cured of H.I.V., Reveals His Identity." *New York Times*, March 9, 2020. https://www.nytimes.com/2020/03 /09/health/hiv-aids-london-patient-castillejo.html.

Mandel, Leah. 2017. "Hurray for the Riff Raff's Video for 'Hungry Ghost' Is a Glowing Ode to DIY Spaces." *The Fader*, January 17, 2017. https://www.thefader.com/2017/01/17/hurray-for-the-riff-raff-hungry-ghost-video.

Martin, Rachel. 2021. "How Families, Separated at the Border by Trump Policies, Are Coping." *NPR*, June 15, 2021. https://www.npr.org/2021/06/15/1006477931/how-families-separated-at-the-border-by-trump-policies-are-coping.

Martínez, Ernesto Javier. 2013. *On Making Sense: Queer Race Narratives of Intelligibility*. Palo Alto, CA: Stanford University Press.

Martínez, Glenn. 2014. "Azucarao: Tato Laviera and the Poetics of Health Promotion." In *The AmeRícan Poet: Essays on the Work of Tato Laviera*, edited by Stephanie A. Alvarez and William Luis, 176–86. New York: CUNY Hunter College Center for Puerto Rican Studies.

Martinez, Monica Muñoz. 2018. *The Injustice Never Leaves You: Anti-Mexican Violence in Texas*. Cambridge, MA: Harvard University Press.

Martínez, Rubén. 2002. *Crossing Over: A Mexican Family on the Migrant Trail*. New York: Picador.

Martinson, Karen Jean. 2005. "Teatro Caliente! (review)." *Theatre Journal* 57, no. 30: 485–89.

McKiernan-González, John. 2012. *Fevered Measures: Public Health and Race at the Texas-Mexico Border, 1848–1942*. Durham, NC: Duke University Press.

McRuer, Robert. 2006. *Crip Theory: Cultural Signs of Queerness and Disability*. New York: New York University Press.

McRuer, Robert. 2010. "Disability Nationalism in Crip Times." *Journal of Literary and Cultural Disability Studies* 4, no. 2: 163–78.

Menchaca, Megan. 2019. "The 'Fattest' City in the U.S. Is in Texas, List Says." *Austin American-Statesman*, March 20, 2019. https://www.statesman.com/story/news/2019/03/20/fattest-city-in-us-is-in-texas-list-says/5665348007/.

Mendoza, Mary E. 2017. "La Tierra Pica/The Soil Bites: Hazardous Environments and the Degeneration of Bracero Health, 1942–64." In *Disability Studies and the Environmental Humanities: Toward an Eco-Crip Theory*, edited by Sarah Jaquette Ray and JC Sibara, 474–501. Lincoln: University of Nebraska Press.

Menjívar, Cecilia, and Olivia Salcido. 2002. "Immigrant Women and Domestic Violence: Common Experiences in Different Countries." *Gender and Society* 16, no. 6: 898–920.

Metzl, Jonathan M. 2010. "Introduction: Why against Health?" In *Against Health: How Health Became the New Morality*, edited by Jonathan M. Metzl and Anna Kirkland, 1–11. New York: New York University Press.

Metzl, Jonathan M. 2019. *Dying of Whiteness: How the Politics of Racial Resentment Is Killing America's Heartland*. New York: Basic Books.

Milian, Claudia. 2019. *LatinX*. Minneapolis: University of Minnesota Press.

Minet, Carla. 2019. "Maria's Death Toll: On the Crucial Role of Puerto Rico's Investigative Journalists." In *Aftershocks of Disaster: Puerto Rico before and after the Storm*, edited by Yarimar Bonilla and Marisol LeBrón, 73–79. Chicago: Haymarket Books.

Mingus, Mia. 2011. "Changing the Framework: Disability Justice." *Leaving Evidence* (blog), February 12, 2011. https://leavingevidence.wordpress.com/2011/02/12/changing-the-framework-disability-justice/.

Minich, Julie Avril. 2014. *Accessible Citizenships: Disability, Nation, and the Cultural Politics of Greater Mexico.* Philadelphia: Temple University Press.

Minich, Julie Avril. 2016. "The Decolonizer's Guide to Disability." In *Junot Díaz and the Decolonial Imaginary: Critical Essays,* edited by Monica Hanna, Jennifer Harford Vargas, and José David Saldívar, 49–67. Durham, NC: Duke University Press.

Minich, Julie Avril. 2017. "Aztlán Unprotected: Reading Gil Cuadros in the Aftermath of HIV/AIDS." *GLQ* 23, no. 1: 167–93.

Mizelle, Richard M., Jr. 2020. "Hurricane Katrina, Diabetes, and the Meaning of Resiliency." *Isis* 111, no. 1: 120–28.

Mizelle, Richard M., Jr. 2021. "Diabetes, Race, and Amputations." *Lancet* 397, no. 10281: 1256–57.

Molina, Natalia. 2006. *Fit to Be Citizens? Public Health and Race in Los Angeles, 1879–1939.* Berkeley: University of California Press.

Molina, Natalia. 2014. *How Race Is Made in America: Immigration, Citizenship, and the Historical Power of Racial Scripts.* Berkeley: University of California Press.

Monteagudo, Jesse. 1995. "Doomsday Spirituality." *Lambda Book Report* 4, no. 8: 34.

Montes, Amelia M. L. 2015. "Creating Art from Diabetes: An Interview with ire'ne lara silva on *enduring azucares.*" *La Bloga* (blog), July 5, 2015. https://labloga.blogspot.com/2015/07/creating-art-from-diabetes-interview.html.

Montes, Amelia M. L. 2016. "The Rituals of Health." In *The Routledge Companion to Latina/o Popular Culture,* edited by Frederick Luis Aldama, 256–66. New York: Routledge.

Montoya, Michael J. 2011. *Making the Mexican Diabetic: Race, Science, and the Genetics of Inequality.* Berkeley: University of California Press.

Moraga, Cherríe, and Gloria Anzaldúa, eds. 1983. *This Bridge Called My Back: Writings by Radical Women of Color.* 2nd ed. New York: Kitchen Table, Women of Color Press.

Morales, Iris. 2016. *Through the Eyes of Rebel Women: The Young Lords: 1969–1976.* New York: Red Sugarcane.

Morales Trujillo, Hilda. 2010. "Femicide and Sexual Violence in Guatemala." In *Terrorizing Women: Feminicide in the Américas,* edited by Rosa-Linda Fregoso and Cynthia Bejarano, 127–37. Durham, NC: Duke University Press.

Moran-Thomas, Amy. 2019. *Traveling with Sugar: Chronicles of a Global Epidemic.* Berkeley: University of California Press.

Moya, Paula M. L. 2016. *The Social Imperative: Race, Close Reading, and Contemporary Literary Criticism.* Stanford, CA: Stanford University Press.

Muñoz, Alicia, and Ariana E. Vigil. 2019. "A Journey to/through Family: Nostalgia, Gender, and the American Dream in Reyna Grande's *The Distance between Us.*" *Frontiers* 40, no. 2: 219–42.

Muñoz, José Esteban. 2009. *Cruising Utopia: The Then and There of Queer Futurity.* New York: New York University Press.

Muñoz, Manuel. 2003. *Zigzagger: Stories.* Evanston, IL: Northwestern University Press.

Muñoz, Manuel. 2007. *The Faith Healer of Olive Avenue.* Chapel Hill, NC: Algonquin Books.

Muñoz, Manuel. 2011. *What You See in the Dark.* Chapel Hill, NC: Algonquin Books.

National Domestic Violence Hotline. n.d. "Help for Friends and Family." Accessed March 12, 2020. https://www.thehotline.org/help/help-for-friends-and-family/.

Nazario, Sonia. 2006. *Enrique's Journey: The Story of a Boy's Dangerous Odyssey to Reunite with His Mother.* New York: Random House.

Nazario, Sonia. 2018a. "Do You Care about the Rule of Law? Then Act Like It." *New York Times,* July 11, 2018. https://www.nytimes.com/2018/07/11/opinion/asylum-immigration-trump.html.

Nazario, Sonia. 2018b. "I'm a Child of Immigrants. And I Have a Plan to Fix Immigration." *New York Times,* October 26, 2018. https://www.nytimes.com/2018/10/26/opinion/caravan-migrants-asylum-trump.html.

Nazario, Sonia. 2019a. "Pay or Die." *New York Times,* July 29, 2019. https://www.nytimes.com/interactive/2019/07/25/opinion/honduras-corruption-ms-13.html.

Nazario, Sonia. 2019b. "'Someone Is Always Trying to Kill You.'" *New York Times,* April 5, 2019. https://www.nytimes.com/interactive/2019/04/05/opinion/honduras-women-murders.html.

Nevins, Joseph. 2002. *Operation Gatekeeper: The Rise of the "Illegal Alien" and the Making of the U.S.-Mexico Boundary.* New York: Routledge.

Ngai, Mae M. 2004. *Impossible Subjects: Illegal Aliens and the Making of Modern America.* Princeton, NJ: Princeton University Press.

Nixon, Rob. 2011. *Slow Violence and the Environmentalism of the Poor.* Cambridge, MA: Harvard University Press.

Noe-Bustamante, Luis, Lauren Mora, and Mark Hugo López. 2020. "About One-in-Four U.S. Hispanics Have Heard of Latinx, but Just 3% Use It." *Pew Research Center,* August 11, 2020. https://www.pewresearch.org/hispanic/2020/08/11/about-one-in-four-u-s-hispanics-have-heard-of-latinx-but-just-3-use-it/.

Novack, Sophie. 2019. "Life and Limb: Inside the Rio Grande Valley's Amputation Crisis." *Texas Observer,* March 1, 2019. https://www.texasobserver.org/life-and-limb/.

Novack, Sophie. 2020. "'I Think I'm Gonna Die': Coronavirus Compounds Risk for Dialysis Patients in the Rio Grande Valley." *Texas Observer,* April 6, 2020. https://www.texasobserver.org/coronavirus-rio-grande-valley-dialysis/.

Obama, Barack. 2017. Facebook post. September 5, 2017. https://www.facebook.com/barackobama/posts/10155227588436749.

Olszewski, Lawrence. 2003. "Crossing Vines." *Library Journal,* September 15, 2003, 91.

Ortiz, Ricardo L. 2007. *Cultural Erotics in Cuban America.* Minneapolis: University of Minnesota Press.

Paredez, Deborah. 2017. "Unaccompanied: An Interview with Javier Zamora." *Poets.org,* October 1, 2017. https://poets.org/text/unaccompanied-interview-javier-zamora.

Pelly, Jenn. 2022. "*Life on Earth*: Hurray for the Riff Raff." *Pitchfork,* February 18, 2022. https://pitchfork.com/reviews/albums/hurray-for-the-riff-raff-life-on-earth/.

Peña, Susana. 2013. *¡Oye Loca! From the Mariel Boatlift to Gay Cuban Miami*. Minneapolis: University of Minnesota Press.

Pérez, Daniel Enrique. 2014. "Toward a Mariposa Consciousness: Reimagining Queer Chicano and Latino Identities." *Aztlán: A Journal of Chicano Studies* 39, no. 2: 95–127.

Perez, Domino Renee. 2008. *There Was a Woman: La Llorona from Folklore to Popular Culture*. Austin: University of Texas Press.

Pérez-Torres, Rafael. 2006. *Mestizaje: Critical Uses of Race in Chicano Culture*. Minneapolis: University of Minnesota Press.

Pickens, Therí Alyce. 2019. *Black Madness :: Mad Blackness*. Durham, NC: Duke University Press.

Piepzna-Samarasinha, Leah Lakshmi. 2015. *Dirty River: A Queer Femme of Color Dreaming Her Way Home*. Vancouver, BC: Arsenal Pulp.

Piepzna-Samarasinha, Leah Lakshmi. 2018. *Care Work: Dreaming Disability Justice*. Vancouver, BC: Arsenal Pulp.

Pitts, Andrea J. 2021. *Nos/Otras: Gloria E. Anzaldúa, Multiplicitous Agency, and Resistance*. Albany: State University of New York Press.

Powers, Ann. 2014a. "Hurray for the Riff Raff's New Political Folk." *NPR*, January 23, 2014. https://www.npr.org/sections/therecord/2014/01/22/265039131/hurray-for-the-riff-raffs-new-political-folk.

Powers, Ann. 2014b. "The Political Folk Song of the Year." *NPR*, December 11, 2014. https://www.npr.org/sections/therecord/2014/12/11/370125443/the-political-folk-song-of-the-year.

Powers, Ann. 2017. "Review: Hurray for the Riff Raff, 'The Navigator.'" *NPR Music*, March 2, 2017. https://www.npr.org/2017/03/02/517792966/first-listen-hurray-for-the-riff-raff-the-navigator.

Price, Margaret. 2015. "The Bodymind Problem and the Possibilities of Pain." *Hypatia: A Journal of Feminist Philosophy* 30, no. 1: 268–84.

Puar, Jasbir K. 2017. *The Right to Maim: Debility, Capacity, Disability*. Durham, NC: Duke University Press.

Puga, Ana Elena. 2016. "Migrant Melodrama and the Political Economy of Suffering." *Women and Performance* 26, no. 1: 72–93.

Puga, Ana Elena, and Víctor M. Espinosa. 2020. *Performances of Suffering in Latin American Migration: Heroes, Martyrs and Saints*. New York: Palgrave.

Ramírez, Dixa. 2018. "Violence, Literature, and Seduction." *Avidly*, May 8, 2018. http://avidly.lareviewofbooks.org/2018/05/08/violence-literature-and-seduction/.

Rendell, Joanne. 2003. "A Very Troublesome Doctor: Biomedical Binaries, World-Making, and the Poetry of Rafael Campo." *GLQ* 9, nos. 1–2: 205–31.

Reston, Maeve. 2020. "Florida and Texas Governors Blame Spike in Cases on Increased Testing." *CNN*, June 18, 2020. https://www.cnn.com/2020/06/18/politics/texas-florida-coronavirus-cases-governors/index.html.

Richie, Beth E. 2012. *Arrested Justice: Black Women, Violence, and America's Prison Nation*. New York: New York University Press.

Rodríguez, Daniel A. 2020. *The Right to Live in Health: Medical Politics in Postindependence Havana*. Chapel Hill: University of North Carolina Press.

Rodríguez, Juana María. 2003. *Queer Latinidad: Identity Practices, Discursive Spaces.* New York: New York University Press.

Rodríguez, Juana María. 2014. *Sexual Futures, Queer Gestures, and Other Latina Longings.* New York: New York University Press.

Rodríguez, Juana María. 2020. "Activism and Identity in the Ruins of Representation." In *AIDS and the Distribution of Crises*, edited by Jih-Fei Cheng, Alexandra Juhasz, and Nishant Shahani, 257–87. Durham, NC: Duke University Press.

Rodriguez, Ralph E. 2018. *Latinx Literature Unbound: Undoing Ethnic Expectation.* New York: Fordham University Press.

Rodríguez, Richard T. 2017. "X Marks the Spot." *Cultural Dynamics* 29, no. 3: 202–13.

Rohrleitner, Marion Christina. 2017. "Chicana Memoir and the DREAMer Generation: Reyna Grande's *The Distance between Us* as Neo-colonial Critique and Feminist Testimonio." *Gender and Research/Gender a Výzkum* 18, no. 2: 36–54.

Román, Elda María. 2013. "'Jesus, When Did You Become So Bourgeois, Huh?': Status Panic in Chicana/o Cultural Production." *Aztlán: A Journal of Chicano Studies* 38, no. 2: 11–40.

Román, Elda María. 2017. "Rerouting the Rise: Upward Mobility in Junot Díaz's Fiction." *Symbolism* 17:103–21.

Romo, Vanessa. 2018. "MIT Clears Junot Díaz of Sexual Misconduct Allegations." *NPR*, June 20, 2018. https://www.npr.org/2018/06/20/622094905/mit-clears -junot-diaz-of-sexual-misconduct-allegations.

Ropp, Sarah. 2019. "Troubling Survivorism in *The Bluest Eye*." *MELUS* 44, no. 2: 132–52.

Roth, Benita. 2017. *The Life and Death of ACT UP/LA: Anti-AIDS Activism in Los Angeles in the 1980s and 1990s.* Cambridge: Cambridge University Press.

Ruiz, Matthew Ismael. 2017. "*The Navigator*: Hurray for the Riff Raff." *Pitchfork*, March 15, 2017. https://pitchfork.com/reviews/albums/22955-the-navigator/.

Ruiz, Sandra. 2019. *Ricanness: Enduring Time in Anticolonial Performance.* New York: New York University Press.

Rumbaut, Rubén G. 1997. "Paradoxes (and Orthodoxies) of Assimilation." *Sociological Perspectives* 40, no. 3: 483–511.

Saldaña-Portillo, María Josefina. 2019. "The Violence of Citizenship in the Making of Refugees: The United States and Central America." *Social Text* 37, no. 4: 1–21.

Sandoval, Edgar. 2020. "I Went Home to Texas to Cover the Virus. Then My Family Got It." *New York Times*, July 14, 2020. https://www.nytimes.com/2020/07/14/us /coronavirus-texas-rio-grande-valley-border.html.

Sandoval-Sánchez, Alberto. 2005. "Politicizing Abjection: In the Manner of a Prologue for the Articulation of AIDS Latino Queer Identities." *American Literary History* 17, no. 3: 542–49.

Santiago, Esmeralda. 1997. *América's Dream.* New York: Harper Perennial.

Schalk, Sami. 2018. *Bodyminds Reimagined: (Dis)ability, Race, and Gender in Black Women's Speculative Fiction.* Durham, NC: Duke University Press.

Schalk, Sami. 2022. *Black Disability Politics.* Durham, NC: Duke University Press.

Schalk, Sami, and Jina B. Kim. 2020. "Integrating Race, Transforming Disability Studies." *Signs: A Journal of Women in Culture and Society* 46, no. 1: 31–55.

Schiller, Dane. 2015. "Immigrant Mother Arrested at Gynecologist's Office Draws National Attention." *Houston Chronicle*, September 17, 2015. https://www.houstonchronicle.com/news/houston-texas/houston/article/Immigrant-mother-arrested-at-gynecologist-s-6512587.php.

Schmidt Camacho, Alicia. 2005. "Ciudadana X: Gender Violence and the De-nationalization of Women's Rights in Ciudad Juárez, Mexico." *CR: The New Centennial Review* 5, no. 1: 255–92.

Segarra, Alynda. 2015. "Alynda Segarra's Call to Folk Singers: Fall in Love with Justice." *The Bluegrass Situation*, May 19, 2015. https://thebluegrasssituation.com/read/alynda-lee-segarras-call-folk-singers-fall-love-justice-op-ed/.

Shah, Nayan. 2001. *Contagious Divides: Epidemics and Race in San Francisco's Chinatown*. Berkeley: University of California Press.

Shear, Michael D., Katie Benner, and Michael S. Schmidt. 2020. "'We Need to Take Away Children,' No Matter How Young, Justice Dept. Officials Said." *New York Times*, October 6, 2020. https://www.nytimes.com/2020/10/06/us/politics/family-separation-border-immigration-jeff-sessions-rod-rosenstein.html.

Shelbourne, Mallory. 2017. "Chaffetz: Americans May Need to Choose between iPhone or Healthcare." *Hill*, March 7, 2017. https://thehill.com/homenews/house/322664-chaffetz-americans-may-need-to-choose-between-buying-new-iphone-or-healthcare.

Shilts, Randy. 1987. *And the Band Played On: Politics, People and the AIDS Epidemic*. New York: Penguin.

silva, ire'ne lara. 2016. *Blood Sugar Canto*. Hilo, HI: Saddle Road.

silva, ire'ne lara. 2017. "ire'ne lara silva talks about embodied poetry and writing *Blood Sugar Canto*." *Rogue Agent Journal*, no. 26 (May 2017). http://www.rogueagentjournal.com/issue26.

silva, ire'ne lara. n.d. "ire'ne lara silva's shame: a ghazal in pieces." *Poetry Society of America*. https://poetrysociety.org/features/in-their-own-words/irene-lara-silva-on-shame-a-ghazal-in-pieces.

Simon and Schuster. n.d. "A Dream Called Home." https://www.simonandschuster.com/books/A-Dream-Called-Home/Reyna-Grande/9781501171437.

Solomon, Dan. 2020. "The Rio Grande Valley Is Texas's Coronavirus Hot Spot." *Texas Monthly*, July 24, 2020. https://www.texasmonthly.com/news-politics/rio-grande-valley-texas-coronavirus-hot-spot/.

Sontag, Susan. 2001. *Illness as Metaphor and AIDS and Its Metaphors*. New York: Picador.

Sotomayor, Sonia. 2002. "A Latina Judge's Voice." *Berkeley La Raza Law Journal* 13, no. 87: 87–93.

Sotomayor, Sonia. 2013. *My Beloved World*. New York: Alfred A. Knopf.

Sotomayor, Sonia. 2018. *Turning Pages: My Life Story*. New York: Philomel Books.

Sotomayor, Sonia. 2019. *Just Ask! Be Different, Be Brave, Be You*. New York: Philomel Books.

Stern, Alexandra Minna. 1999. "Buildings, Boundaries, and Blood: Medicalization and Nation-Building on the U.S.-Mexico Border, 1910–1930." *Hispanic American Historical Review* 79, no. 1: 41–81.

Swan, Jonathan. 2017. "Scoop: Trump Privately Predicts He Will Appoint Four Justices." *Axios*, October 15, 2017. https://www.axios.com/scoop-trump-privately-predicts-he-will-appoint-four-justices-1513306203-6274d9b0-1824-45ee-8556-fade9bdb2fd8.html.

Taubes, Gary. 2011. *Why We Get Fat: And What to Do about It.* New York: Anchor Books.

Taubes, Gary. 2016. *The Case against Sugar.* New York: Anchor Books.

Taylor, Sunny. 2004. "The Right Not to Work: Power and Disability." *Monthly Review* 55, no. 10: 30–44.

Thompson, Ginger. 2018. "Families Are Still Being Separated at the Border, Months after 'Zero Tolerance' Was Reversed." *ProPublica*, November 27, 2018. https://www.propublica.org/article/border-patrol-families-still-being-separated-at-border-after-zero-tolerance-immigration-policy-reversed.

Tomso, Gregory. 2004. "Bug Chasing, Barebacking, and the Risks of Care." *Literature and Medicine* 23, no. 1: 88–111.

Tovar, Virgie. 2015. "I'm a Fat Anti-assimilationist (& No I'm Not Sorry)." *virgietovar.com*, July 21, 2015. https://www.virgietovar.com/blog/im-a-fat-anti-assimilationist-no-im-not-sorry.

Treichler, Paula A. 1999. *How to Have Theory in an Epidemic: Cultural Chronicles of AIDS.* Durham, NC: Duke University Press.

Tretheway, Natasha. 2020. *Memorial Drive: A Daughter's Memoir.* New York: Ecco.

United Nations High Commissioner for Refugees. 2004. "UNHCR Letter to Attorney General Relating to the Matter of Rodi Alvarado Peña." January 9, 2004. https://www.refworld.org/docid/43e9f6e64.html.

US Department of Justice. 2018. "Matter of A-B-." 27 I&N Dec. 316 (A.G.).

Vargas, Deborah R. 2016. "Sucia Love: Losing, Lying, and Leaving in Díaz's *This Is How You Lose Her.*" In *This Is How You Lose Her: Junot Díaz and the Decolonial Imagination*, edited by Monica Hanna, Jennifer Harford Vargas, and José David Saldívar, 351–75. Durham, NC: Duke University Press.

Varón, Alberto. 2018. "Introduction: The Places and Spaces of Latinx Cultures." *Chiricú Journal* 3, no. 1: 8–20.

Vázquez, Adela. 2015. "Finding a Home in Transgender Activism in San Francisco." In *Queer Brown Voices: Personal Narratives of Latina/o LGBT Activism*, edited by Uriel Quesada, Letitia Gomez, and Salvador Vidal-Ortiz, 212–20. Austin: University of Texas Press.

Vega, William A., and Hortensia Amaro. 1994. "Latino Outlook: Good Health, Uncertain Prognosis." *Annual Review of Public Health* 15:39–67.

Viego, Antonio. 1999. "The Place of Gay Male Chicano Literature in Queer Chicana/o Cultural Work." *Discourse* 21, no. 3: 111–31.

Villa, Raúl Homero. 2000. *Barrio-Logos: Space and Place in Urban Chicano Literature and Culture.* Austin: University of Texas Press.

Villarosa, Linda. 2022. *Under the Skin: Racism, Inequality, and the Health of a Nation.* London: Scribe.

Viramontes, Helena María. 1985. *The Moths and Other Stories.* Houston, TX: Arte Público.

Viramontes, Helena María. 2007. *Their Dogs Came with Them*. New York: Atria.

Viruell-Fuentes, Edna A. 2007. "Beyond Acculturation: Immigration, Discrimination, and Health Research among Mexicans in the United States." *Social Science and Medicine* 65, no. 7: 1524–35.

Viruell-Fuentes, Edna A., Patricia Y. Miranda, and Sawsan Abdulrahim. 2012. "More than Culture: Structural Racism, Intersectionality Theory, and Immigrant Health." *Social Science and Medicine* 75, no. 12: 2099–106.

Wald, Priscilla. 2008. *Contagious: Cultures, Carriers, and the Outbreak Narrative*. Durham, NC: Duke University Press.

Wald, Sarah D. 2016. *The Nature of California: Race, Citizenship, and Farming since the Dust Bowl*. Seattle: University of Washington Press.

Wanzer-Serrano, Darrel. 2015. *The New York Young Lords and the Struggle for Liberation*. Philadelphia: Temple University Press.

Ward, Anna E. 2013. "Fat Bodies/Thin Critique: Animating and Absorbing Fat Embodiments." *S&F Online* 11, no. 3. https://sfonline.barnard.edu/life-un-ltd -feminism-bioscience-race/fat-bodiesthin-critique-animating-and-absorbing -fat-embodiments/.

Wear, Delise, and Julie M. Aultman. 2005. "The Limits of Narrative: Medical Student Resistance to Confronting Inequality and Oppression in Literature and Beyond." *Medical Education* 39, no. 10: 1056–65.

White House. 2009. "Remarks by the President to a Joint Session of Congress on Health Care." September 9, 2009. https://obamawhitehouse.archives .gov/video/President-Obama-Address-to-Congress-on-Health-Insurance -Reform#transcript.

Wilhelm, Robert. 2010. "Delia's Gone, One More Round." *Murder by Gaslight* (blog), March 21, 2010. http://www.murderbygaslight.com/2010/03/delias-gone -one-more-round.html.

Wilkerson, Abby L. 2012. "Normate Sex and Its Discontents." In *Sex and Disability*, edited by Robert McRuer and Anna Mollow, 183–207. Durham, NC: Duke University Press.

Woodruff, Judy, and Amna Nawaz. 2019. "Kirstjen Nielsen on Trump's Controversial Immigration Policies and Why She Resigned." *PBS NewsHour*, October 22, 2019. https://www.pbs.org/newshour/show/kirstjen-nielsen-on-what-she -regrets-about-her-tenure-at-dhs.

Zamora, Javier. 2017. *Unaccompanied*. Port Townsend, WA: Copper Canyon.

Zamora, Javier. 2022. *Solito: A Memoir*. New York: Penguin Random House.

INDEX

curative violence, 16, 140
Cutler, John Alba, 13
Cvetkovich, Ann, 55, 58, 140

Dalleo, Raphael and Elena Machado
  Sáez, 110
Daniels, Caitlin, 69–70
Danticat, Edwidge, 147–48
Davis, Lennard, 168n3
de Burgos, Julia, 153
Dean, Tim, 32–33
debility, 3, 129
Decena, Carlos Ulises, 27, 171n10
Decolonize Your Diet, 177n25
Deferred Action for Childhood Arrivals
  (DACA), 2, 117–18, 142
Deferred Action for Parents of Americans
  and Lawful Permanent Residents
  (DAPA), 118
Delacre, Lulu, 61
"Delia's Gone" (song), 94, 179n9
DeSantis, Ron, 20
diabetes, 9–11, 19, 22, 51, 53–55, 57–68, 70–81,
  174n1, 174n2, 176n11, 176n12, 177n23,
  177n24, 178n2
Diabetic Sugar Slam, 66
diagnosis, 34, 50, 54, 59, 68, 76, 140, 145,
  158–59
dialysis, 53, 55
Díaz, Junot, 23, 119–20, 127–30, 133–35,
  140–41, 148, 183n10, 183n11, 183n12,
  183n13
Diedrich, Lisa, 45, 48, 173n22
disability, 4–6, 8–10, 12–13, 15–17, 22, 31,
  54–55, 62, 64, 74–75, 82–85, 129–30,
  140, 146, 156–62, 168n2, 168n3, 170n14,
  176n12, 178n2; disability justice, 5, 16,
  82–83, 114, 155; disability rights, 4–5, 13;
  disability studies, 3–4, 6, 19, 21–3, 114,
  133, 157–59, 161, 168n4; and race, 4, 129,
  168n4; medical model of, 3
domestic abuse, 22; 81; 83; 85; 87; 89; 92–93;
  103; 107–8; 112–13; 125; 128; 177n1;
  178n2. *Consult also* violence
Dominican Republic, 108–12, 132, 135
DREAM Act, 124; DREAMer, 118, 142–43
Dugas, Gaëta, 50, 174n26
Dunn, Timothy, 182n7
Duvalier, François, 148

eczema, 16–17
Edelman, Lee, 118, 182n6
Edinburg, TX, 52, 117n21
Eils, Colleen Gleeson, 103
El Salvador, 90, 135–41, 183n16
Ellis, Amanda, 71, 74, 174n1
Ellis Island, 5
empathy, 15, 45, 48, 83, 90, 102–07, 173n22,
  178n5
Ensler, Eve, 67–68, 177n20
Erevelles, Nirmala, 9, 13
Esperanza Peace and Justice Center, 67

Farabundo Martí National Liberation Front
  (FMLN), 183n16
Farber, Jim, 94
fat, 9, 12, 56–57, 61, 68, 73, 75, 161, 177n21;
  fatness, 9–10, 56, 73; fatphobia, 161
feminicide, 87, 91–92, 178n3; feminicidal vio-
  lence, 86–87, 91, 178n3; feminicidio, 87
feminist, 3, 82–84, 86–87, 92, 94, 102, 129,
  133, 144, 151, 153, 162, 178n3
feminist-of-color disability studies, 4
Ferguson, Roderick A., 4
Fielding-Singh, Priya, 69–70, 177n22
Figueroa-Vásquez, Yomaira C., 128, 135
Fisher, Gary, 46–47
Flores, Juan, 64
Freeman, Gregory, 171n9
Fregoso, Rosa-Linda, 83–84, 86–87, 107
Fregoso, Rosa-Linda and Cynthia Bejarano,
  87
Fresno, 98–99
Fulton, Sybrina, 96, 180n12

García, Patricia M., 122
García-Peña, Lorgia, 108
Garden, Rebecca, 105
Garland, Merrick, 179n7
Gay Men's Health Crisis (GMHC), 173n17
Gay, Roxane, 86
Gil'Adi, Maia, 128–29, 183n11
Gilmore, Leigh, 105
Gilmore, Ruth Wilson, 3
González, Isabel, 5, 8, 168n4
González, Octavio R., 171n10
González, Rigoberto, 22, 84, 87–88, 102–7,
  112, 181n17
Gordon, Colin, 8–9; 169n9